HIDDEN *Healing* POWERS
of
SUPER & WHOLE
FOODS

PLANT-BASED DIET PROVEN TO PREVENT & REVERSE DISEASE

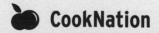 CookNation

HIDDEN *Healing* POWERS OF SUPER & WHOLE FOODS

PLANT-BASED DIET PROVEN TO PREVENT & REVERSE DISEASE

ISBN 978-1-912155-88-0
Cover image under license from Shutterstock
Printed and bound by CPI Group (UK) Ltd, Croydon, CRO 4YY

Disclaimer

Except for use in any review, the reproduction or utilisation of this work in whole or in part in any form by any electronic, mechanical or other means, now known or hereafter invented, including xerography, photocopying and recording, or in any information storage or retrieval system, is forbidden without the permission of the publisher.

This book is sold subject to the condition that it shall not, by way of trade or otherwise, be lent, resold, hired out or otherwise circulated without the prior consent of the publisher in any form of binding or cover other than that in which it is published and without a similar condition, including this condition being imposed on the subsequent purchaser.

This book is designed to provide information on plant-based ingredients and their believed benefits. This information is provided and sold with the knowledge that the publisher and author do not offer any legal or other professional advice.

In the case of a need for any such expertise consult with the appropriate professional.

This book does not contain all information available on the subject, and other sources of recipes are available.

Every effort has been made to make this book as accurate as possible. However, there may be typographical and/or content errors. Therefore, this book should serve only as a general guide and not as the ultimate source of subject information.

This book contains information that might be dated and is intended only to educate and entertain.

The author and publisher shall have no liability or responsibility to any person or entity regarding any loss or damage incurred, or alleged to have incurred, directly or indirectly, by the information contained in this book.

— Contents —

Healing Fruit

Healing Nuts & Beans

Healing Herbs 69

4-Week Food Diary 86

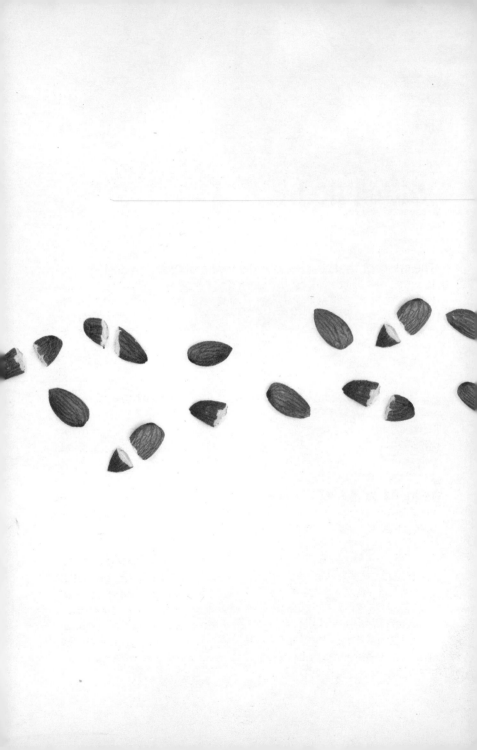

Introduction

The concept that diet is essential to the prevention and treatment of ailments was first widely accepted thanks to Hippocrates - the ancient Greek physician now regarded as the father of medicine. Hippocrates is credited with removing the superstition and intervention of gods surrounding medicine and instead, collected data based on experiments. He is famously quoted as saying

"Let food be thy medicine and medicine be thy food".

He recognised the importance and effect of diet on our health and his advice was to focus on nutrients from food as a means of preventing and treating disease.

Thankfully our scientific understanding of food has come a long way since ancient Greek times, but the idea of healing oneself by using food as medicine remains the same.

This book aims to list many of the greatest plant-based healing food and offer a layman's guide to how and why they can help with your overall wellbeing. The Hidden Healing Powers of Super & Whole Foods documents food according to their known and believed health benefits. Each food listed will enlighten you to its potential benefits and aims to change the way you perceive fruit, vegetables, nuts, beans and herbs. They are a life-giving source of nutrition and energy.

The human body, by design, is built to survive. It knows to regenerate cells, to remove toxins and with its inbuilt immune system, to fight disease and illness. To perform these daily tasks it must of course receive fuel. The fuel that we give our bodies needs to contain the correct micro and macronutrients so that it can keep us healthy. While the advance of medical science continues to grow, no medical practitioner or scientist will ever disagree that preventative medicine should always be the first step to a healthier life. The intervention of modern drugs has undoubtedly eased the suffering of millions on a daily basis and for this we should of course be grateful. However we all too often overlook the natural ways in which we can feed our bodies with healing properties.

While super and whole foods can help relieve the symptoms of many minor ailments such as headaches or skin irritations, they can also be instrumental in fighting some of the worlds biggest killers, such as diabetes and heart disease - both of which are highly influenced by diet. The health benefits of fruit and vegetables are well documented. We are told on a daily basis to eat more of them in order to create a healthy balanced diet. For years now government-initiated campaigns to push the 5-a-day fruit & veg message to young children and their parents has become something that will all know to be beneficial to our health, yet most of us fail to achieve this daily quota for ourselves and our families.

Despite the proven rich health benefits of eating more fruit and vegetables, in our modern world of fast food and convenience their appeal remains low. In order to truly appreciate fruit, vegetables,nuts and herbs we must understand and appreciate them not just as '5-a-day necessities' but as powerful, healing, disease-preventing miracles that come from the earth, are inexpensive and readily available to all of us and easy to include in our diet every day. By changing the way we perceive plant-based foods and their hidden healing powers they suddenly no longer become a bore, a chore or something that *should* be eaten, when in reality we'd rather eat something else. Instead we see them a in a new light. A light which shines brightly on the long list of health benefits that could help us manage problematic ailments, low moods and stave off life- threatening diseases.

For example, *kale*, while a good source of protein can also help with depression.
It contains omega-3 acids, iron, folate and vitamin B6 which all contribute to making serotonin and dopamine to elevate mood. The presence of copper also helps boost the immune system and creation of more blood cells.

Apricots have a number of qualities, including high levels of calcium that helps to maintain strong bones. They are also a great source of fibre, which can help relieve constipation and maintain a healthy bowel.

When we understand and appreciate these incredible benefits, how can we not fully embrace their power, while not forgetting the amazing taste they bring into our meals? There are thousands of different ways we can prepare, cook and present plant-based foods to make them exciting and tasty - that's a whole other book; The purpose of this guide is to open our eyes to the life-changing benefits and hidden healing powers of super and whole foods.

This book does not in any way seek to challenge or conflict with medical science or man-made drugs and intervention, but instead aims to enlighten us all to the innumerable benefits that naturally-grown plant life can give us.

At the end of this book you will also find a 4-week food diary. Food diaries are an indispensable way of accurately analysing what we eat. Often it is not until we can see what we eat each

day written down that we realise how much of it is unhealthy and how much it could be improved. You may find at a glance how lacking in plant-based foods your diet actually is.
For those who may feel like they suffer from a food intolerance, keeping a food diary is an excellent way to begin the process of identifying and eliminating any potential foods that may be the cause of symptoms linked to an intolerance.

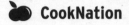 **CookNation**

HIDDEN *Healing* POWERS

of
FOODS

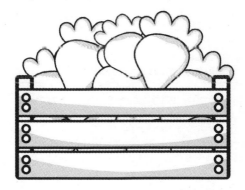

Aloe Vera

- **Aloe Vera can make your skin glow and hair glossy**
  It is full of vitamins and minerals that bring a healthy, natural glow to your skin and hair.
- **Aloe Vera can reduce indigestion**
  Boasting an impressive range of fatty acids, Aloe Vera contains components that help reduce acid indigestion, which is also linked to reducing allergic reactions and food intolerances.
- **Aloe Vera is good for your heart**
  Aloe Vera contains HCL Cholesterol, a fatty acid that lowers the amount of fat in the blood. Whilst it will not undo a poor diet, nor compete with the benefits exercise brings to the heart, Aloe Vera can reduce your cholesterol to an extent.
- **It boosts your immune system**
  Aloe Vera is recognised as an 'Adaptogen'; an Adaptogen is something that helps our bodies to, quite literally, adapt. This takes form in enabling the body to adapt more easily to changes, building resilience and boosting the immune system to fight off illness. Rather than reaching for the cough mixture or Lemsip when you are next unwell, try some Aloe Vera instead.
- **It can help irritable bowel syndrome (IBS).**
  As well as reducing indigestion, Aloe Vera helps with digestion. It can help regulate your bowels to help with diarrhoea, constipation and IBS.
- **Aloe Vera helps to detox the body**
  Aloe Vera is referred to as a 'gelatinous food'. When consumed, as gelatinous foods move through our bodies, they absorb toxins which then exit the body through our 'waste', cleansing the intestinal system and detoxing the body.
- **It works as an anti-bacterial agent.**
  Aloe Vera contains a number of active ingredients, such as sulphur and nitrogen, which help prevent the growth of bacteria. But, unlike many products bought in stores, Aloe Vera acts as an anti-bacterial naturally, rather than containing harsh chemicals.
- **Aloe Vera can reduce scarring and stretch marks**
  Due to its healing nature and qualities as an Adaptogen, using the gel of Aloe Vera has been cited by many as an effective way of reducing the appearance of scars and stretch marks with, in some cases, dramatic changes reported.

Artichoke

- **Artichokes can fight anaemia**
  Rich in iron, artichokes help the production of red blood cells and can combat the negative symptoms associated with anaemia and formation of the iron deficiency.
- **Artichokes can help prevent diabetes**
  Artichokes, through their high fibre content, are able to facilitate the maintenance of stable blood sugar levels as well as reducing insulin resistance, since glucose is absorbed more slowly.
- **Artichokes may prevent cancer**
  Numerous antioxidants and phytonutrients are found in artichokes, including rutin and quercetin, which can help reduce the damage caused by free radicals, fight oxidative stress and limit cancerous and pre-cancerous cell growth.
- **Artichokes for detoxification**
  Artichokes are known to promote the production of bile and healthy bacteria in the digestive system, facilitating the detoxification of the liver and digestive system and promoting healthy function.
- **Artichokes promote healthy skin**
  Antioxidants and essential vitamins and minerals are all found in artichokes and contribute to healthy skin through preventing gaining, promoting hydration and maintaining the structure of the skin's layers.
- **Artichokes can aid weight loss**
  High levels of soluble fibre are present in artichoke, which has been correlated with maintaining a healthy weight and helping you lose weight as they fill you up and curb your appetite.
- **Artichokes promote a healthy cardiovascular system**
  Regularly ingesting artichokes has been associated with reducing the ratio of bad to good cholesterol in the body, increasing blood flow and fighting inflammation, all of which are preventative for cardiovascular diseases.
- **Artichokes help lower blood pressure**
  Due to the high amount of potassium in artichokes, it has been suggested that they act as vasodilators and can reduce blood pressure through neutralising the levels of sodium in the body.
- **Artichokes can help the digestive system**
  High in fibre, artichokes can help the digestive system work more efficiently and relieve issues such as constipation, inflammation and cramps.

Asparagus

- **Asparagus removes excess fluid**
  It is a natural diuretic and increases production of urine in the body, eliminating extra fluid. This is important for individuals who suffer from a build up of water, known as edema, or who have a high blood pressure.
- **Asparagus helps healthy bones**
  Rich in Vitamin K, Asparagus is an essential nutrient in enabling the body to absorb calcium. Through increasing calcium absorbance, the risk of osteoporosis is reduced.
- **Asparagus is an antioxidant**
  High in antioxidants, including anthocyanins, which protect the body through the prevention of inflammation and reducing the damage caused by free radicals.
- **Asparagus promotes digestive health**
  Both soluble and insoluble fibres are found in artichokes, both of which are essential in maintaining regular bowel movement, digestive health and relieving constipation.
- **Asparagus supports cardiac health**
  Vitamin K, found in asparagus, is a blotted clotting vitamin that supports a number of cardiac functions and prevents the hardening of arteries; it is also associated with lowering the risk of cardiovascular diseases.
- **Asparagus for pregnancy**
  High concentrations of folate, found in asparagus, are very important for rapid gestation during pregnancy and folate has been linked to a reduced risk of pregnancy complications, defects and miscarriage.
- **Asparagus boosts immunity**
  Vitamin E is an important antioxidant contained in asparagus that plays a key role in protecting the body from free radical damage and facilitates the functioning of your immune system, helping you fight off infections.
- **Asparagus for sexual stamina**
  Asparagus is a natural aphrodisiac as it contains vitamin B6 and folate, known to boost arousal, and vitamin E that stimulates the production of sex hormones oestrogen and testosterone.

Aubergine

- **Aubergine helps lower cholesterol**
  Evidence indicates that consumption of eggplant juice can significantly lower the levels of bad cholesterol in your blood, as it contains chlorogenic acid.
- **Aubergines boost cognition**
  Nasunin is an anthocyanin in the skin of aubergines and has strong antioxidant properties that protect the brain from free radical damage, as well as reducing neuroinflammation.
- **Aubergines support your heart**
  Aubergines contain fibre, vitamin C, potassium and vitamin B6, all of which contribute to maintaining a healthy heart. It has also been associated with a reduced risk of heart disease.
- **Aubergines may be anti-carcinogenic**
  Due to the high levels of polyphenols in aubergine, such as chlorogenic acid and anthocyanin, it is believed that it may have anti-cancer effects through preventing cancer cell growth and reducing inflammation.
- **Aubergines help improve digestion**
  Aubergines are a natural source of both soluble and insoluble fibre, which aid in digestive health and regular bowel movements as well as increasing the absorption of nutrients throughout the digestive tract.
- **Aubergines support your bones**
  Phenolic compounds, found in aubergine, have been associated with the strengthening of bones, increased bone density and a reduced risk of developing osteoporosis.
- **Aubergines aid weight loss**
  The low fat content and high levels of fibre present in aubergine make them an ideal food for weight loss as they are nutritious and the fibre fills you up and can suppress your appetite.
- **Aubergines combat anaemia**
  Aubergines contain high levels of iron and also copper, which facilitate the healthy maintenance of red blood cells, helping to combat anaemia.
- **Aubergines can boost your energy levels**
  High in iron, aubergines can provide you with a health boost of energy when consumed as part of a balanced diet.

Beetroot

- **Beetroot may fight dementia**
  Research has shown that drinking beetroot juice can increase blood oxygen levels in the brain, which slows the progression of dementia. and may prevent premature age-related decline in cognitive function.
- **Beetroot reduces inflammation**
  Beetroot contains the essential nutrient choline, which can aid maintenance of cell membranes and the reduction of inflammation that is often associated with chronic diseases.
  Beetroot lowers blood pressure
  Evidence has shown that beetroot juice lowers your blood pressure due to its high content of nitrates that dilate blood vessels and increase blood flow.
- **Beetroot may be anti-diabetic**
  Alpha-lipoic acid is an antioxidant found in beetroot, which has been shown to reduce glucose levels and promote insulin sensitivity, with it being suggested as an ideal food for reducing the symptoms associated with diabetes.
- **Beetroot boosts physical performance**
  Juice extracted from beetroot has been shown to have vasodilation properties, which improve the transport of oxygen to muscles when exercising, boosting your energy for a better workout or performance.
- **Beetroot may prevent cancer**
  Betanin, found in beetroot, may potentially be preventative for several cancers including prostrate, lung and breast cancer, as it can decrease the proliferation of cancer cells.
- **Beetroot facilitates digestion**
  Red beetroots are often used to relieve constipation and treat other digestive complaints, as they are rich in fibre and also improve blood supply to the digestive system.
- **Beetroot supports liver function**
  Beetroot contains calcium, B vitamins, iron, antioxidants and betaine, all of which contribute to a healthy liver function.
- **Beetroot can help a hangover**
  Beetroot also thins bile and helps eliminate toxins, further enhancing liver function and helping your body to recover from alcohol consumption and/or poisoning.

Broccoli

- **Broccoli strengthens your bones**
  High levels of vitamin K, concentrated in broccoli, are essential in facilitating calcium absorption and increasing bone density, with adequate intake being linked to a decreased risk for osteoporosis.
- **Broccoli for detoxification**
  Broccoli contains vitamin and sulphur, both of which are well known detoxifiers that aid in the elimination of toxins from the body and fight the damage caused by free radicals.
- **Broccoli is anti-aging**
  Vitamin C is an antioxidant found in broccoli that can prevent the signs of aging by reducing skin damage, keeping the skin hydrated and also maintaining a healthy structure of collagen in the skin layers.
- **Broccoli may prevent cancer**
  Ingesting a high amount of cruciferous vegetables, including broccoli, has been linked to a reduced risk of both lung and colon cancers. Research suggests this is due to them containing sulforaphane, an inhibitor of cancer cell growth.
- **Broccoli provides protection from UV**
  Glucoraphanin is a phytonutrient found in broccoli and evidence suggests that is can reverse some of the damage caused by exposure to UV rays from the sun.
- **Broccoli improves vision**
  Several compounds known to play a role in maintaining eye health, including vitamin A, beta-carotene and phosphorus, are found in broccoli. Research has shown they can protect the eyes from macular degeneration and are associated with delaying the development of cataracts.
- **Broccoli for Amyotrophic Lateral Sclerosis (ALS)**
  Studies have shown that foods rich in omega-3 fatty acids, such as broccoli, could potentially delay the onset of the neurodegenerative disorder ALS.
- **Broccoli can boost your energy levels**
  High in iron, Broccoli can give you a healthy and sustained boost to your energy levels, increasing your red blood cell count.
- **Broccoli is good during pregnancy**
  Pregnant women are more susceptible to iron deficiencies, such as anaemia, and so eating iron-rich foods, such as broccoli, can help prevent such deficiencies and maintain energy levels.

Carrots

- **Carrots improve ocular health**
  Carrots are a rich source of the antioxidant beta-carotene and vitamin A; both have been associated with improved vision, reduction of night-blindness and a reduced risk of macular degeneration.
- **Carrots regulate your sugar levels**
  High levels of carotenoids, present in carrots, have been associated with a reduced risk of diabetes as they can decrease insulin resistance and lower blood sugar levels. Additionally, they facilitate in the metabolism of insulin and glucose in the body.
- **Carrots can boost immunity**
  Numerous antiseptic, antibacterial compounds and a high level of vitamin C is found in carrots, which makes them the perfect food to boost the immune system and help fight infection.
- **Carrots may prevent strokes**
  Evidence suggests that a regular intake of carrots can reduce your risk of stroke due to the presence of beta-carotene. Moreover, in one study, beta-carotene levels were positively correlated with survival rate in stroke patients.
- **Carrots help oral health**
  Several mineral antioxidants are found in carrots that can stimulate the production of saliva, which fights the bacteria in oral cavities and reduces bad breath and the risk of tooth decay.
- **Carrots aid digestion**
  Carrots are rich in dietary fibre, which is essential in maintaining a healthy digestive system through regular bowel movements and can be used to relieve constipation and reduce inflammation of the gut.
- **Carrots can make your skin glow**
  Rich in Vitamin A and C, amongst many other nutrients, carrots can help give your skin a natural glow and improve its general appearance.
- **Carrots can help you keep a tan**
  Carrots contain Beta Carotene which cannot necessarily make you tan better, but it can help you maintain a tan and healthy glow for longer.
- **They can help with weight loss**
  The fibre in carrots, and their low calorie content, make them a perfect alternative snack that keeps you fuller for longer, helping with weight loss and general weight management.

Cauliflower

- **Cauliflower is anti-inflammatory**
  Evidence suggests that foods high in fibre could fight inflammation and lower the risk of many diseases associated with chronic inflammation, such as cardiovascular disease and autoimmune diseases.

- **Cauliflower improves digestion**
  Due to the high water and fibre content of cauliflower, it is effective in maintaining a healthy digestive system, preventing constipation and possibly lowering the risk of colon cancer as toxins are eliminated more frequently.

- **Cauliflower boosts cognitive function**
  Choline, found in cauliflower, is an essential compound that has been shown to facilitate sleep, memory, and learning, as it helps neuronal transmission and can reduce neuroinflammation.

- **Cauliflower aids healthy circulation**
  Plenty of dietary fibre has been shown to reduce the risk of cardiovascular diseases resulting from poor circulation as it prevents the build-up of calcium in the blood vessels

- **Cauliflower may prevent cancer**
  Cauliflower contains several antioxidants that can reduce the damage caused by free radicals and oxidative stress. One such antioxidant, indole-3-carbinol, has been associated with a decreased risk for reproductive cancers as it may prevent cell mutations and uncontrolled growth.

- **Cauliflower aids hormonal balance**
  Antioxidant rich foods, such as cauliflower, aid in maintaining a healthy hormonal balance in the body, through reducing excessive levels of oestrogen.

- **Cauliflower aids weight loss**
  Cauliflower is a low calorie, high fibre food with a high water content, all of which contribute to weight loss as they are filling and can supress appetite. Also, cauliflower can serve as a substitute for some high calorie foods, including rice and flour.

- **Cauliflower improves vision**
  Sulforaphane, present in cauliflower, is a nitrate that has been shown to protect retinal tissue from oxidative stress and UV damage, as well as helping maintain healthy ocular functions.

Cabbage

- **Cabbage is good for your brain**
  Vitamin K and anthocyanins help with concentration and mental function. Cabbage - especially red cabbage - can help protect you from dementia and other neurodegenerative diseases.
- **Cabbage can help prevent cancer**
  Lupeol, sinigrin and sulforaphane are all found in cabbage and can stimulate enzyme activity while inhibiting cell mutations and destroying free radicals, which can help prevent the development of cancer.
- **For headaches**
  For chronic headaches, drinking raw cabbage juice can help alleviate the symptoms.
- **Skin**
  Cabbage helps with acne-prone skin, using sulfur to make keratin, necessary for healthy nails, skin and hair.
- **Weight control**
  Cabbage is high in fibre and low in fat. It can support the digestive system as well as help detoxify the body. Vitamin C helps get rid of free radicals and uric acid.
- **Bone strength**
  Vitamins C and K help protect our body from free-radical damage, as well as boosting the immune system. Vitamin K keeps bones strong and healthy, reducing the risk of osteoporosis.
- **Cholesterol**
  Cabbage can help to reduce absorption of fat by bile after a meal. This lowers cholesterol levels in the body
- **Sore muscles**
  Cabbage is a source of lactic acid when fermented, which can help with sore muscles when applied as a compress.

Celery

- **Weight loss**
  Celery is low in calories and contains fibre, which helps to make you feel full for longer.
- **Hydration**
  Being about 95% water, celery is a good way of keeping up fluid levels, especially during the summer months.
- **Good for cholesterol levels**
  Celery fibres pick up excess cholesterol and encourages elimination. The compound phthalide reduces bad cholesterol and blood pressure.
- **Pheromones**
  Celery contains high levels of the male hormones androstenone and androstanol, which could potentially increase men's attractiveness and boost arousal levels.
- **Eye care**
  One stalk of celery provides 5% of the daily Vitamin A intake, which prevents degeneration of vision.
- **Cancer combat**
  Flavonoids in celery help to inhibit cancer cell growth, especially in the pancreas and the formation of breast cancer cells.
- **Digestion**
  Anti-inflammatory properties of celery can help protect the digestive tract. Apiuman found in celery has shown properties leading to improvement of the stomach lining and decreased risk of stomach ulcers.
- **Liver health**
  Experiments have shown a reduction of fat buildup in the liver from celery in the diet. Celery also helps improve liver enzyme function.
- **UTIs**
  Due to its effects on uric acid and high water content, celery is good at fighting bacterial infections of the digestive and reproductive organs. This also helps protect from kidney problems and cysts.

Courgette

- **Helps you lose weight**
  Courgettes are low in calories but have the power to satisfy your appetite. They are also rich in fibre and water.
- **Courgette improves eye health**
  Courgette can help to remove puffy bags under your eyes, as well as enhance vision due to its vitamin A content.
- **Courgette for cholesterol**
  Using vitamins A and C, courgettes can delay atherosclerosis and reduce cholesterol. It also helps to remove excess toxins and its anti-inflammatory properties can help protect against diabetes.
- **Courgettes contain antioxidants**
  Antioxidants help to reduce brain cell degeneration. Vitamin E and Omega 3 fatty-acids help stimulate their absorption.
- **Courgettes for men's health**
  Courgettes in the diet show promising results in decreasing symptoms of Benign Prostatic Hypertrophy, helping resolve sexual and urinary problems.
- **Cardiovascular system**
  Courgettes contain manganese and vitamin C which help to maintain strong heart health. It helps to decrease blood pressure and the build-up of cholesterol through the electrolyte potassium interacting with and balancing sodium.
- **Important for healthy DNA**
  Courgettes contain folates, which help with DNA synthesis and cell division. Therefore, it can also help prevent neural defects in foetuses.
- **B-complex**
  Courgettes contain some B-complex vitamins, which all help maintain a healthy cell metabolism.

Edamame

- **Vitamin boost**
  A half-cup serving of edamame contains 10% of the daily value of vitamins A and C. It is also high in iron, good for preventing anaemia.
- **Cholesterol regulation**
  Regular soy food consumption helps to regulate cholesterol levels, preventing the development of atherosclerosis. Isoflavones in beans also work to protect against cancer and osteoporosis.
- **Skin health**
  Antioxidants in edamame help to repair damaged skin and maintain its health. Isovflavones also help here as they may be involved in managing age-related skin changes.
- **Edamame for lung health**
  Genistein, an isoflavone in the beans, may be beneficial for asthma sufferers. Genistein also affects uncontrolled cell growth in cancer and vascular inflammation seen in atherosclerosis.
- **Edamame protein source**
  Due to its protein content, edamame helps to maintain healthy muscle mass. Folate and Vitamin K support a healthy heart. It can be a protein source for vegetarians, at the same time enhancing cardiovascular benefits.
- **Reduced risk of osteoporosis**
  Due to its calcium content, edamame reduces the risk of weak bones, by increasing the bone-mineral density, especially in older women.
- **Edamame for breast cancer risk**
  Edamame can help reduce the risk of breast cancer, which is seen in Asian women who consume it in high amounts.
- **Edamame and infants**
  Edamame can be successful in treating infants with lactose intolerance. It can also help reduce diarrhoea.

Kale

- **Kale for depression**
  Eating kale benefits good mircoorganisms found in our gut,
  maintaining a healthy digestive system. It also contains omega-3
  acids, protein, iron, folate and vitamin B6 which all contribute to
  making serotonin and dopamine to elevate mood.
- **Good for diabetics**
  Kale contains sulforaphane which helps control blood sugar levels.
  Other players such as Vitamins C, K and A as well as beta-carotene
  and manganese also help turn proteins into sugar.
- **Immunity boost**
  Kale contains 10% of the recommended daily intake of copper, which
  helps boost your immune system and the creation of more blood
  cells.
- **Magnesium for metabolism**
  Magnesium found in kale stimulates 300 enzyme reactions in the
  body, it is important for nutrient metabolism and energy creation.
- **Kale for cancer**
  Kale contains organosulfur compounds that help break down cancer
  cells. These compounds also boost the immune system, overall
  working to maintain a healthy body to fight against cancer.
- **Detoxify**
  Kale can help detoxify your body as it contains fibre and sulphur,
  which help to maintain liver health and function.
- **Filled with antioxidants**
  Kale is loaded with antioxidants, which mop up free radicals in the
  body, protecting us from atherosclerosis, cognitive decline and
  inflammation.
- **Healthy pregnancy**
  Kale is nutrient-dense and iron is especially useful during pregnancy.
  A good amount of iron in the diet helps protect the foetus from low
  birth weight or premature birth or its consequences.

Leek

- **Cardiovascular support**
  Leeks contain flavonoid kaempferol, which helps protect blood vessels from damage. Folate in leeks also supports the cardiovascular system by keeping amino acids in balance.
- **Leeks contain Allicin**
  Allicin is a sulphur-containing compound which has anti-bacterial, anti-viral and anti-fungal properties, as well as the power to neutralise free radicals.
- **Leeks for digestion**
  Leeks contain prebiotics, which are good bacteria that helps the gut work and stay healthy. These also eliminate toxic waste and improve digestive function.
- **Leeks for healthy cholesterol**
  Leeks can decrease bad cholesterol (LDL) in the blood and increase the levels of good cholesterol (HDL).
- **Leeks for anaemia**
  The iron found in leeks helps prevent anaemia, and along with its vitamin C content, it can improve iron absorption.
- **Pregnancy and leeks**
  Leeks contain folate which is important for healthy foetal development
- **Weight loss**
  Leeks are low in calories and contain fibre, which helps to fill your stomach and also boosts metabolism. They are also good for your skin due to vitamin C and A, along with various antioxidants. They can contribute to sun protection and detoxification.
- **Leeks for the eyes**
  Leeks can also improve vision, using lutein and zeaxanthin to filter our harmful rays which can lead to harmful DNA oxidation. These can also protect from cataracts and macular degeneration.

Mushroom

- **Mushrooms for the immune system**
  Protein, fibre, B vitamins and antioxidants all help to prevent damage to cells. Mushrooms contain natural antibiotics that help protect against infections and aid ulcer healing.
- **Mushrooms for cholesterol**
  Mushrooms could help lower cholesterol, which in turn protects the heart by keeping a healthy blood pressure.
- **Cancer**
  Some mushroom varieties have shown cancer-protecting properties, by protecting from DNA damage. They could also be beneficial in the treatment or management of neurodegenerative diseases.
- **Increase vitamin D**
  The only fruit or vegetable that contains vitamin D, mushrooms help with the absorption of vital minerals and maintain healthy biological processes.
- **Mushrooms and inflammation**
  Mushrooms have anti-inflammatory properties, helping to fight disease, suppress allergic symptoms and even reduce tumour growth
- **Mushrooms for ageing**
  A recent study has shown the potential for anti-ageing properties of mushrooms. They contain antioxidants ergothioneine and glutathione, which display such assets.
- **Mushrooms rich in selenium**
  Selenium is typically found in animal proteins, therefore mushrooms can help vegetarians obtain the correct amounts of this protein. It benefits bone health, increasing strength, as well as strengthening teeth, hair and nails. Selenium also helps fight free radicals to strengthen the immune system.

Onion

- **Immunity**
  Phytochemicals and vitamin C help to boost the immune system
- **Blood sugar**
  Onions contain chromium, which works to regulate blood sugar levels. This can be beneficial for diabetics. The combination of biotin and chromium might help regulate blood sugar levels
- **Cholesterol**
  Onions lower the presence of bad cholesterol (LDL) in the blood, helping to maintain a healthy heart
- **Anti-cancer**
  Onions contain quercetin, which has been known to play a role in preventing cancer. It also contains potent antioxidants, which help get rid of free radicals and prevent cell death.
- **Stings**
  Applying onion to stings reduces burning and pain, giving immediate relief. Onions show anti-inflammatory and anti-bacterial properties
- **Healthy skin**
  Biotin found in onions is important for maintenance of healthy nails, hair and skin.
- **Digestion**
  Onions contain fibre, which helps maintaint a healthy digestive system. Menopausal women showed a 20% decrease in risk of health disease when incorporating onions into their diet.
- **Cure for fever**
  Onions can be mixed with other health foods, such as honey, to alleviate symptoms of common cold, fever or allergies.
- **Onion for teeth**
  Raw onions can improve oral health by eliminating bacteria, helping maintain healthy gums and teeth.

Pea

- **Antioxidant and anti-inflammatory properties**
  Peas contain catechin and epicatechin as well as carotenes, all work to lower risk of heart disease, type II diabetes and arthritis.
- **Good for diabetics**
  Green peas provide us with fibre and protein that help regulate digestion. They can lower fasting blood sugar as well as insulin levels
- **Good for bones**
  Peas contain a good amount of vitamin K, which increases calcium absorption by bones. This also helps prevent osteoporosis
- **Cholesterol**
  Niacin found in peas helps lower the level of bad cholesterol (LDL) and increase good cholesterol (HDL)
- **Good for a healthy stomach**
  Peas contain coumestrol, which has been effective in helping prevention of stomach cancer.
- **Prevents anaemia**
  Peas are loaded with iron, which helps prevent fatigue and other symptoms of anaemia. The vitamins also help to boost your energy levels.
- **Reduces depression**
  Peas help to reduce the effects of depression, through the folate found in them. The antioxidants present also contribute to lowering depression and mood swings.
- **Learning enhancement**
  The vitamin thiamine is important for increasing energy , focus and improving memory.
- **Ageing**
  Peas help to prevent the signs of ageing. The antioxidants present help to reduce free radical damage as well as help clear toxins, which in turn make you feel healthier and younger.

Radish

- **Weight loss**
  Radishes are filling but low in carbohydrates, and also contain a lot of water. They also contain a lot of fibre, which helps regulate bowel movements and the efficiency of metabolism.
- **Leucoderma - loss of skin pigment**
  Radish seeds can help to detoxify the body and aid treatment of skin disease.
- **Blood pressure**
  Radishes are a source of potassium, which helps reduce blood pressure, relax blood vessels and increase blood flow. This also contributes to maintaining a healthy heart
- **Good for kidneys**
  Radishes are a diuretic and disinfectant and can help treat kidney disorders by aiding in detoxification.
- **For bites**
  Radishes are anti-pruritic and can reduce pain and swelling after an insect bite.
- **Liver and Gallbladder protection**
  Radishes help to regulate bile production and other liver enzymes. They also help to remove excess bilirubin from the blood, protecting your liver from damage.
- **Asthma**
  Radishes show anti-congestive properties, which can help to fight allergies and regulate the respiratory system, protecting delicate membrane lining.
- **Skin benefits**
  Radishes also help to keep not only the body but also the skin hydrated, due to their high water content. This slows down skin ageing and wrinkles, helping to maintain healthy skin.

Raw Honey

- **Raw honey can prevent hayfever**
  Consuming one teaspoon of raw honey a day can dramatically reduce or prevent reactions for hayfever sufferers. The raw honey must be sourced from as local a producer as possible for it to take affect and needs to be consumed for a few months prior to 'hayfever season' to allow your body to build up a barrier to your local pollen.

- **It is a healthy alternative to sugar**
  Honey is naturally sweet and is frequently used as an alternative to sweeteners. However, sweetened honey may not be any better than sugar. Raw honey can add a little bit of sweetness with no negative effects and can help stabilise blood sugar levels.

- **It is good for spots!**
  Whether you suffer from the odd pimple or more severe acne, raw honey is great for healing skin conditions, minimising infection through stopping bacteria growth and minimising any associated odours from such conditions.

- **Raw honey can boost your energy levels**
  Raw honey is mainly formed of natural sugar, which means it can be more easily absorbed (unlike unnatural sugars), making it perfect for an energy boost to kick start your morning or exercise routine.

- **It can clear up your cough**
  Raw honey has been used for decades, if not centuries, as a natural way to soothe a sore throat, reduce mucus, and clear up a traditional cough and cold without the need for medicine.

- **Raw honey can reduce the risk of cancer**
  Full of antioxidants, raw honey contains polyphenol and pinocembrin. Polyphenol is a powerful antioxidant that has been shown in studies to reduce the risk of cancer and heart disease; pinocembrin is also a powerful antioxidant that helps the body to initiate killing off specific cells that may be of threat to the body, including certain cancer cells.

- **It makes you sleep better**
  Raw honey releases nutrients into your body which help your brain and body remain balanced and therefore reduces the chance of you being awoken in the night by your brain.

- **Raw honey is a natural antibacterial agent**
  Ideal for healing cuts and wounds, raw honey is full of goodness that prevents bacteria growing in the area to which it is applied, making it a wonderful natural antibacterial agent.

Salad Greens

- **Good for your eyes**
  Carotenoids such as vitamin A help eyes adapt from bright light to darkness. Lutein also helps filter out high-energy light, protecting eyes from damage.
- **Heart protection**
  Salad greens contain folate and fibre which lower the risk of stroke and cardiovascular disease. These can also reduce levels of bad cholesterol (LDL)
- **Diabetes**
  Salad greens are rich in magnesium which can help lower the risk of Type II diabetes and help control insulin resistance.
- **Easy sleep**
  Lettuce contains lactucarium which has been used to treat sleep problems such as insomnia, as the compound can help induce sleep
- **Good for muscles**
  Salads contain nitrates, which boost the production of certain proteins that make muscles stronger and more efficient.
- **Antioxidants**
  Antioxidants found in salads help to reduce the risk of heart ailments, improve circulation in the body and boost the immune system
- **Weight loss**
  Low in calories, you can eat salad greens as part of any diet. Fibre gives you the 'full' feeling, as it inhibits the release of a hormone which makes you hungry. In turn this can reduce snacking and overeating.

Spirulina

- **Spirulina is great for vegans or vegetarians**
  Spirulina is a phenomenal source of protein; some report that up to 70% of spirulina is actual, natural protein. It acts as a brilliant supplement but does come at a high cost.
- **Spirulina is just as nutritious as milk**
  It most certainly does not come from a cow; however, spirulina is said to contain as much calcium and magnesium as found in cow's milk.
- **It can help your eyesight and improve brain activity**
  Spirulina makes waves in the superfood market, due to it containing vitamin B12; a lack of B12 in the body has been linked to deterioration of the brain and eyesight, as well as general mental health issues, such as depression.
- **Spirulina can help digestion**
  When ingested, as spirulina passes through the body, it absorbs toxins that we do not want nor need, and acts as a detoxifier, improving digestion and liver and bowel movements.
- **Spirulina can reduce allergies**
  It is believed that spirulina can help reduce some reactions to allergies, such as sneezing, itchiness and a runny nose. This is because it is thought to prevent histamines from being released into the body, which is what initiates the reactions in the first place.
- **Spirulina can help with memory retention**
  As well as containing B12 to help prevent brain deterioration, spirulina is also believed to prevent oxidative damage, otherwise known as memory loss. You just need to remember to take it.
- **It could replace cholesterol medication**
  Whilst spirulina cannot solve the underlying issues that cause high cholesterol, it is believed to effectively reduce cholesterol levels as a natural alternative to medication.
- **Spirulina can help fight cancer**
  In particular, the consumption of spirulina has been linked to effective reduction and/or treatment of oral cancers. Studies showed that a daily controlled consumption of spirulina led to a regression of pre-cancerous and cancerous lesions in the mouth in 45% of patients.
- **It boosts your immune system**
  Full of nutrients and antioxidants, spirulina can boost your immune system and help your body to fight off common coughs, colds and viral infections.

Sprout

- **Good for your heart**
  Sprouts contain omega-3 fatty acids, which form good cholesterol. They also reduce cardiovascular stress, while potassium reduces blood pressure.
- **Sprouts for pregnancy**
  Sprouts are rich in folate, which helps prevent neural tube defects.
- **Anti-cancer**
  Vitamins C, A and proteins help to eliminate free radicals in the body, preventing cell mutations. The organic compounds present can also have positive effects on cognitive decline and other age-related health issues.
- **Allergies**
  Some varieties of sprout can help reduce allergic reactions and inflammatory response.
- **Colds**
  Lysine, an enzyme found in sprouts, can help remove cold sores and boost your immune system
- **Hair benefits**
  Sprouts contain selenium, which is a fungus that helps to remove dandruff. It also stimulates hair growth and relieves symptoms of itchy scalp
- **Hormones**
  Sprouts can help to correct hormonal imbalances, which can affect a variety of things such as mood, fertility and even hair loss.
- **Good for acne**
  Consuming sprouts can give you healthy, smooth skin, with reduced inflammation from acne or psoriasis.

HIDDEN *Healing* POWERS

of

FRUIT

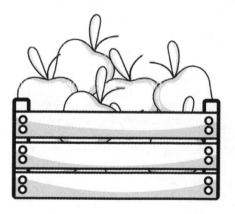

Apple

- **Apples have antioxidant effects**
  Apples are rich in essential antioxidants, phytonutrients and flavonoids, and these may reduce your risk of hypertension, heart disease and diabetes.
- **Apples are great for digestion**
  As the apple peel contain lots of dietary fibre, when eaten they aid with digestive and bowel movements and also help in maintaining healthy cholesterol levels.
- **Apples can improve neurological health**
  Quercetin is one of the many antioxidants found in apples, which has been found to reduce inflammation and cell death in the brain leading to a healthier brain.
- **Apples improve your memory**
  Consuming apple juice has been shown to increase the levels of the neurotransmitter acetylcholine, an important chemical for the functioning of the brain, improving memory and reducing the risk of Alzheimer's disease.
- **Apples support your immune system**
  Vitamin C is a powerful antioxidant, naturally found in apples, that has been shown to block toxic free radicals and also increase the body's resistance to infection.
- **Apples help maintain a healthy nervous system**
  Several B-complex vitamins are found in apples, which play a key role in maintaining red blood cells and cells of the nervous system
- **Apples protect your body from free radical damage**
  Polyphenolic compounds naturally occur in apples and have been shown to help protect your body from the effects of free radicals and environmental toxins. These compounds have also been shown to help reduce the risk of several inflammatory diseases.
- **Apples improve oral health**
  As eating an apple stimulates your mouth to produce more saliva, this decreases the level of bacteria in your mouth and can reduce the risk of tooth decay leading to whiter and healthier teeth.
- **Apples may help fight against cancer**
  There are high levels of flavonol in apples, a compound that is thought to have cellular anti-growth properties and has been linked to a reduced risk of developing several types of cancers, including breast, colon and pancreatic cancer.

Apricot

- **Apricots improve eyesight**
  Rich in Vitamin A, apricots can help improve your eyesight and decrease your risk of developing serious eye and vascular diseases.
- **Apricots fight earache**
  The oil from apricots can be dropped into your ear canal and this has been shown to be a rapid and effective treatment for earaches due to the anti-inflammatory properties of apricots.
- **They boost your immune system**
  Rich in nutrients and vitamins, apricots boost your immune system helping your body to naturally fight off illness.
- **Apricots relieve constipation**
  As they are high in fibre, it is thought apricots are an effective way of combating constipation and maintaining healthy bowel movements.
- **Apricots improve cardiac health**
  The high fibre content of apricots has also been shown to reduce the levels of bad cholesterol and increase the levels of good cholesterol in your blood, protecting your heart and reducing the risk of cardiovascular diseases.
- **Apricots toughen your bones**
  Apricots contain high levels of calcium, an essential mineral in the development of bones and maintenance of good bone density, and have been shown to decrease your risk of osteoporosis.
- **Apricots boost your metabolism**
  Due to the high fibre and mineral content of apricots, it has been suggested that they can boost the rate of your metabolism by improving your digestive health.
- **Apricots help relieve asthma**
  The oil extracted from apricots has been shown to have anti-asthmatic qualities and aid in relieving stress and pressure on the respiratory system, helping prevent asthma attacks and boost lung function.
- **Apricots treat anaemia**
  As apricots contain high levels of iron and copper, they can boost the levels of haemoglobin in your blood and help reduce the fatigue associated with anaemia.
- **Apricots can give you clear skin**
  With high levels of both Vitamin A and C, Apricots, have antioxidant properties and help in replacing dying skin cells leading to a slowing of the skin ageing process.

Avocado

- **Avocados are great for digestion**
  High in fibre, avocados can have great benefits on your digestive system helping to reduce inflammation and cramping

- **Avocados can help diabetics**
  Avocados help to control, steady and maintain blood sugar levels, which can be of great benefit to sufferers of diabetes.

- **They help to protect your eyes**
  Two phytochemicals, zeaxanthin and lutein, are found in avocados and protect your eyes from the damage of light, including ultraviolet.

- **Avocados help fight cancer**
  They are high in folate, a vitamin that is thought to prevent cell mutations and is associated with a decrease in risk for many cancers

- **Avocados are beneficial for your skin**
  The monosaturated fats contained in avocados are essential in maintaining moisture levels in the layers of your skin, making it feel soft and look healthy.

- **Avocados can help skin pigmentation**
  Omega-9 fats found in avocados can reduce skin irritation and redness, as they help to repair damaged cells.

- **Avocados promote healthy pregnancy**
  High in folate, avocados contribute to a healthy pregnancy, foetus and neural development.

- **Avocados are great for your heart**
  Avocados contain an abundance of good fats that help lower cholesterol levels, reducing inflammation and blood pressure which decreases the risk of heart and vascular disease.

- **Avocados can help combat depression**
  High in folate, consuming avocados can reduce the risk of developing depression, as they enable the correct delivery of essential nutrients to the brain and help maintain the level of important mood chemicals in the brain, including dopamine and serotonin.

- **Avocados for arthritis treatment**
  The high levels of several nutrients found in avocados, including monosaturated fats, Vitamin C, Vitamin E, carotenoids, and antioxidants, have been shown to decrease the inflammation in the body that is involved in the development of arthritis.

Banana

- **Bananas boost your energy**
  Bananas are said to be a powerhouse of nutrients for your body, as they are packed full of vitamins and minerals, including calcium, potassium, iron, niacin and B6, all of which lead to a healthy functioning of the body.
- **Bananas are full of potassium**
  Due to a high content of potassium, bananas have several benefits, as this mineral is involved in the regulation of blood pressure, cardiac function, electrolyte balance and brain alertness.
- **Bananas are good for digestion**
  Foods rich in fibre, such as bananas, are great for bowel movements and relieving constipation. Additionally, bananas are prebiotic and promote the growth of friendly bacteria in the gut and bowel.
- **Bananas help control blood sugar levels**
  Bananas contain an insoluble fibre called pectin and soluble resistant starch, both of which are known to help control blood sugar after meals, as they lead to a gradual and prolonged release of sugar, rather than a fast spike in sugar levels.
- **Bananas promote natural healing**
  As bananas are high in antioxidants, such as catechines, which protect the body from the damage of free radicals and inflammation.
- **Bananas can help reduce morning sickness**
  High in potassium, it is believed that bananas can help ease nausea and morning sickness and restore your electrolyte balance.
- **Bananas are good for a fever**
  Rich in antioxidants, bananas have been shown to help lower your body temperature when experiencing a fever in illness
- **Bananas improve kidney function**
  Potassium is an essential vitamin for maintaining healthy kidney function and a low blood pressure, with a diet high in potassium being linked to a decreased risk in developing kidney disease or cancer.
- **Bananas are great for fitness**
  High in nutrients, bananas are easily digested and can reduce muscle cramps, soreness and fatigue following exercise.
- **Bananas help fight anaemia**
  High in iron, bananas are great for sufferers of anaemia and aid fatigue, paleness and shortness of breath associated often experienced by anaemics.

Blackberries

- **Blackberries help brain performance**
  Rich in nutrients and antioxidants, blackberries are great for brain function, with benefits including reduced inflammation, increased short-term memory, attention and motor skills, and a possible protective agent for neurodegeneration.
- **Blackberries may help fight cancer**
  They contain flavonoids and lignans, which may aid in the fight against cancer as they can slow cellular growth and are also recommended as a chemotherapeutic.
- **Blackberries can boost your immune system.**
  Blackberries are high in nutrients that support your immune system and have antioxidant and antibacterial properties against harmful toxins.
- **Blackberries aid digestion**
  Blackberries are high in both soluble and insoluble fibre which are vital in helping the digestive system function properly.
- **Blackberries can help weight management**
  Blackberries have a very low fat and sugar content, making them a perfect snack alternative to aid weight loss or maintain a healthy weight.
- **Blackberries are good for your heart**
  Blackberries contain flavonols, fibre and magnesium, all of which have been shown to aid smooth blood flow and prevent arteries from being blocked, helping you maintain a healthy heart. These components have also been linked to a reduced risk of strokes and cardiovascular disease.
- **They can help prevent you ageing**
  Blackberries are high in Vitamin E, which prevents wrinkles from forming, while Vitamin C keeps the skin toned and protects from toxic UV damage.
- **Blackberries aid diarrhoea**
  It is believed that blackberry leaves are effective in treating diarrhoea, as the astringent tannins have healing properties, especially when ingested.
- **Blackberries promote menstrual health**
  Vitamin K in blackberries helps in the clotting of your blood and aids hormone function. It is believed that blackberries can also relieve period pain.

Blueberries

- **Blueberries are anti-ageing**
  Blackberries are high in antioxidants, in particular proanthocyanidins, which has been shown to have anti-ageing properties as well as reduce inflammation and stress.
- **Blueberries support digestive health**
  Blueberries are a great source of both soluble and insoluble fibre, which help maintain regular bowel movements and relieve bowel irritation or constipation.
- **They can improve cognition**
  Blueberries are rich in phenols, such as gallic acid, which is believed to be a superfood for the brain, helping boost performance and memory.
- **Blueberries are great for healthy skin**
  Studies suggest that blueberries help regulate your hormone levels and can help fight acne, additionally they contain an agent, resveratrol, which has been proven to protect against the damage of overexposure to the sun.
- **Blueberries may protect against cancer**
  High in antioxidants, blueberries can reduce the oxidative DNA damage and inflammation that is associated with several chronic illnesses, including cancer. Through neutralising the free radicals that cause this damage, Blueberries may be protective against several cancers.
- **Blueberries aid weight loss**
  Blueberries are naturally high in fibre, low in calories and low on the glycaemic index, making them an ideal food when losing weight.
- **Blueberries lower your blood pressure**
  As blueberries are very low on the glycaemic index it has been suggested that they increase the ratio of good to bad cholesterol in the body and lower blood pressure.
- **They can help prevent heart attacks**
  Since blueberries can help cholesterol and blood pressure levels, it is thought that regular ingestion of blueberries can prevent hypertension and heart attacks.
- **Blueberries are an anti-diabetic**
  Blueberry juice and extract have been shown to have anti-diabetic effects on glucose metabolism and insulin sensitivity, which is associated with a reduced risk of type II diabetes.

Cherries

- **Cherries are an antioxidant**
  Powerful antioxidants, including cyaniding and anthocyanins, are found in cherries and are known to reduce inflammation and the damage caused by free radicals.
- **They help maintain your nervous system**
  Rich in many antioxidants, cherries can help maintain a healthy, functioning nervous system.
- **Cherries help you sleep**
  Cherries contain melatonin, which plays a vital role in your sleep cycle; increasing your intake of melatonin can help you sleep and improve the length and quality of your sleep.
- **Cherries are neuroprotective**
  Due to the antioxidant compounds found in cherries, regular ingestion has been linked to improved memory and cognitive function, with the possibility of them protecting against neurodegeneration, including Alzheimer's.
- **Cherries promote cardiac health**
  Anthocyanins are antioxidants found in cherries that give them their red colour. Research suggests that these compounds activate PPAR, which is a key player in regulating genes necessary for fat and glucose metabolism, leading to cardiovascular benefit and a reduced risk for high blood pressure and stroke.
- **Cherries can help fight gout**
  It is thought that cherries may neutralise the auto-inflammatory nature of gout, an arthritic condition, reducing the pain and risk of attacks.
- **Cherries are anti-ageing**
  It has been said that cherries contain the highest level of antioxidants out of all of the fruits, and cherry juice has been shown to slow down the ageing process of the skin and also boost immunity, helping it to fight free radicals and pathogens.
- **Cherries can help weight loss**
  Cherries are a high fibre snack with a low glycaemic index, with evidence suggesting that cherry ingestion can reduce the levels of bad fat in the blood, reduce your percentage of fat mass and reduce fat from abdominal areas.

Chillies

- **Chillies are powerful antioxidants**
  They are high in antioxidants, which have been linked to protecting the body from free radical damage and inflammation.
- **Chillies boost your immune system**
  High in Vitamin C, consuming chillies can give your immune system a brilliant boost.
- **They can maintain your youth**
  Vitamin C, which is found in chillies, is an essential vitamin for producing and maintaining collagen in the body, helping to maintain skin elasticity and a youthful appearance.
- **Chillies improve circulation**
  It has been suggested that chillies, through reducing the amount of fibrin in your blood, act as blood thinners, which can boost your circulation, improve your cardiac health and be protective against strokes.
- **Chillies are decongestants**
  Ingesting chillies causes your nasal passages to dilate, which allows you to breathe more easily.
- **Chillies aid fat burn**
  Capsaicin, found in chillies, is a thermogenic compound that has been shown to increase your metabolic rate and hence speed up the rate at which your body burns fat.
- **Chillies can help relieve pain**
  The main bioactive compound found in chillies is capsaicin and it has been shown to bind to pain receptors and desensitise them to some types of pain, including heartburn and migraines.
- **Chillies can reduce inflammation**
  Capsaicin is said to contain a neuropeptide that is involved with inflammatory processes in the body. Evidence has shown that ingesting chillies regularly can reduce the symptoms of some auto inflammatory diseases including arthritis and rheumatism.
- **Chillies help reduce blood sugar levels**
  Although it is not yet clear how, research has shown that regularly eating chillies significantly controls your insulin levels after eating and this reduction in insulin sensitivity may reduce the symptoms of diabetes and lower the risk of developing type II diabetes.

Coconut

- **Coconut aids digestion**
  As raw coconut is packed with dietary fibre, it is great for adding bulk to your stool, maintaining bowel movements and being effective at relieving constipation.
- **Coconut may protect from cancer**
  Due to a reduction in insulin and the removal of free radicals from the body, it has been suggested that coconut may be a protective agent against cancer.
- **Coconut boosts energy levels**
  Coconuts are a good natural source of energy and have been suggested as a perfect food for athletes due to high levels of potassium, which can help restore electrolyte balance after a workout.
- **Coconut supports your kidneys**
  Research suggests that ingesting coconut is effective in protecting against bladder infections and kidney diseases.
- **They are great for your skin**
  Coconut creams and oils can effectively hydrate your skin making it silky soft and helping with dryness
- **Coconut boosts the immune system**
  It has been claimed that several components of coconuts, including caprylic and lauric fatty acids, have antibacterial, antifungal and antiviral properties, of which help support the immune system in fighting toxins, infection and disease.
- **They help you heal**
  The antibacterial qualities of coconuts can help your body naturally heal itself, making them great for body cleanses.
- **Coconut protects your heart**
  As coconut contains healthy fats, it increases the ratio of good to bad cholesterol in your body, thus improving blood pressure and acting as a protective agent for heart disease.
- **Coconut prevents tooth decay**
  The oil from a coconut has antibacterial properties that can fight the bacteria that builds up and cause tooth decay.
- **Coconut stabilises blood sugar**
  The high fibre and healthy fat content of raw coconut promotes the slow release of sugar and lowering of blood pressure, both of which are vital in maintaining healthy levels of blood sugar and are protective against diabetes and hypertension.

Cranberries

- **Cranberries can support your cardiovascular system**
  Cranberries contain numerous anti-inflammatories and antioxidants, which can help prevent cardiovascular diseases.
- **Cranberries are good for urinary infections**
  Urinary tract infections (UTIs) are common in women and are caused by pathogens, including E-coli. It is believed that drinking cranberry juice can prevent these infections from occurring and lead to reduced levels of harmful bacteria in the urinary tract.
- **Cranberries can help fight cancer**
  It is believed that cranberries may help in the prevention of several cancers, though possibly inhibiting cellular growth preventing the growth of tumours.
- **They can help bad breath**
  Cranberries contain proanthocyanidins which can prevent bacteria from binding to your teeth and give you fresher breath
- **Cranberries can reduce the risk of gum diseases**
  In addition to reducing breath odours, cranberries can also help reduce the risk of gum disease because of their high antioxidant content.
- **Cranberries are anti-ageing**
  Due to the high presence of antioxidants and phytonutrients in cranberries, they may have a therapeutic effect in protecting cells from the free radical damage that can contribute to ageing.
- **Cranberries help beat the common cold**
  High in antioxidants, cranberries can boost your immunity and fight off the common cold
- **They are an antiseptic**
  Benzoic acid, one of many antioxidants found in cranberries, has strong antiseptic properties and has been linked with a reduced risk of infections and viruses as it can attack pathogens.
- **Cranberries can help you detox**
  It is believed that cranberries have cleaning, antiseptic, detoxifying and diuretic properties, which are ideal for cleansing your body.
- **They can help with digestion**
  The antioxidant and diuretic qualities of cranberries, can all help balance the levels of good and bad bacteria in your digestive tract, as well as flushing harmful toxins out of your body and facilitating regular bowel movements.

Cucumber

- **Cucumbers are high in antioxidants**
  High levels of antioxidants, such as vitamin C, beta-carotene and flavonoids, can reduce the build up of toxic free radicals that are associated with several diseases and chronic illnesses.
- **Cucumbers help relieve stress**
  Cucumbers are packed full of numerous B vitamins, including B5, B7 and B1, all of which are known to reduce feelings of anxiety and also fight the physical damage of stress on the body.
- **Cucumbers are neuroprotective**
  Fisetin, an anti-inflammatory flavonol, is found in cucumbers and plays an essential role in brain health. Specifically, fisetin can improve your memory and act as a protective factor against age-related degeneration and the associated diseases.
- **Cucumbers are hydrating**
  Cucumbers consist of around 95% water and for this reason they can keep your body well hydrated when eaten.
- **They are great for your metabolism**
  Water accounts for a high proportion of the make up of cucumbers which, when consumed, can therefore increase your metabolic rate.
- **Cucumbers are great for detoxing.**
  Low in calories, but high in water and antioxidants, cucumbers are great for flushing toxins out of the body.
- **Cucumbers support digestion**
  Due to the high water and fibre content of cucumbers, ingestion can help food move through your digestive system more quickly and promote regular bowel movements, as well as helping alleviate both acid reflux and constipation.
- **Cucumbers benefit your hair and nails**
  Silica, a mineral contained in cucumber, is known to make both your hair and nails stronger and shinier. Chilled cucumber on the eyes can also help reduce puffiness and redness.
- **Cucumbers control blood sugar**
  Animal research has shown that cucumbers can reduce blood sugar levels and help maintain blood sugar at a healthy level, possibly being able to prevent complications related to diabetes and lowering the risk of developing type II diabetes.

Dates

- **Dates alleviate constipation**
  High in fibre, dates are great for your digestive system and bowel movements, helping to ease constipation, cramps and inflation.
- **Dates help lower your cholesterol**
  Dates are very low in fats and free from cholesterol, with evidence suggesting that they facilitate the maintenance of a healthy ratio of good to bad cholesterol in the body.
- **Dates strengthen your bones**
  Several essential minerals are found in dates, including copper, manganese, magnesium and selenium. All of these are involved in developing and maintaining healthy and strong bones.
- **Dates are anti-inflammatories**
  High levels of magnesium are present in dates, a mineral known for its anti-inflammatory effects. Evidence has shown that regular intake of magnesium can lower the risk of developing cardiovascular disease, Alzheimer's disease and arthritis.
- **Dates boost cognition**
  Vitamin B6, found in dates, has been associated with an improved cognitive and memory performance in several studies.
- **Dates can treat anaemia**
  Rich in iron, dates are an ideal snack for those suffering from anaemia as increasing your iron intake can lead to decreased fatigue and increased strength, due to more red blood cells being produced.
- **Dates cure allergies**
  Dates naturally contain organic sulphur, an element that has been shown to be effective in reducing allergic reactions and lowering the occurrence of seasonal allergies.
- **Dates support your nervous system**
  The high quantities of potassium in dates promote a healthy nervous system, as potassium is a key player in maintaining electrolytes as part of a responsive nervous system and may also increase brain alertness.
- **Dates can increase sexual functioning**
  Dates are known to be a natural aphrodisiac and studies suggest that ingesting them can increase your sex drive and also increase sexual endurance in males.

Figs

- **Figs support your digestive system**
  The very high concentration of fibre in figs adds bulk to your stools and promotes regular bowel movements, aiding in the alleviation of constipation and prevention of diarrhoea.
- **Figs can prevent heart disease**
  Phenol, omega-6 and omega-3 fatty acids are all contained in figs and are known to inhibit triglycerides and reduce the risks of coronary and other heart diseases.
- **They may help fight respiratory conditions**
  The leaves of figs contain natural compounds that can be consumed in a tea for the treatment of numerous respiratory conditions, including asthma and bronchitis.
- **Figs stabilise blood glucose**
  Research has shown that fig leaves can reduce the levels of glucose in the blood and that they may be a treatment for diabetes, as they also have antioxidant properties, which can reduce the oxidative stress caused by diabetes.
- **They can help with acne**
  Because of the high levels of antioxidants in figs, consuming them has shown to help reduce the appearance of acne and prevent the condition from worsening
- **Figs may prevent colon cancer**
  The high amount of fibre that figs provide is essential in maintaining regular bowel movements and ensuring that toxins are removed from your digestive system. Mucin is another compound found in figs that helps eliminate waste from the body,
- **Figs can lower cholesterol**
  Several compounds found in figs, including omega fatty acids, phytosterols and the insoluble fibre pectin, are known to lower cholesterol levels in the body through reducing the natural synthesis of cholesterol and aiding the elimination of any excess cholesterol.
- **Figs strengthen your bones**
  Calcium, potassium, and magnesium are minerals found in figs, which facilitate bone development and help maintain healthy bone density and strength through protecting against age-related breakdown.

Goji Berries

- **Goji Berries boost the immune system**
  High levels of Vitamin C and A are found in goji berries, both of which are essential to maintain immune function and help fight common colds and infections

- **They help fight chronic illnesses**
  Packed with nutrients, goji berries not only boost your immune system, but they also help to reduce inflammation in the body with most chronic illnesses.

- **Goji berries are powerful antioxidants**
  Goji berries are considered a superfood due to the numerous antioxidants they contain, including carotenoids, Vitamin C and zeaxanthin, which protect against free radicals.

- **Goji berries are good for your skin**
  Beta-carotene is concentrated in goji berries and is known to repair damage to the skin, for example from UV light, and promote healthy, clear skin with it being associated with a reduced risk for developing skin cancer.

- **Goji berries help with weight loss**
  Due to the low sugar and high fibre content of the goji berry, this makes them an ideal fruit for snacking and eating healthily and aiding with weight loss.

- **They suppress sweet cravings**
  Goji Berries make you feel fuller for longer and can therefore help to suppress cravings for sweet foods.

- **Goji Berries keep your eyes healthy**
  Antioxidant compounds found in Goji berries, such as zeaxanthin, help improve vision and prevent damage to the eyes from oxidative stress and age-related diseases.

- **Goji berries help regulate blood sugar**
  Goji berries contain very little sugar and a high amount of fibre, which can contribute to the lowering of blood sugar levels and potentially can reduce insulin resistance, both of which are risk factors in type II diabetes.

- **Goji berries improve liver function**
  Some research has suggested that the antioxidant properties of goji berries can protect the liver from free radical damage and help facilitate detoxification of the liver.

Grapefruit

- **Grapefruit helps with weight loss**
  It is one of the lowest calorie fruits yet is still high in nutritional value and fibre content, making it a facilitator of weight loss and management as part of a healthy diet.
- **Grapefruit prevents insulin resistance**
  Research has shown that grapefruit can control insulin levels in the body and are associated with a reduced risk of developing resistance to insulin.
- **Grapefruit is a powerful antioxidant**
  Vitamin C, lycopene, flavanones and beta-carotene are all antioxidants found in grapefruits that provide numerous health benefits, as they protect your body from free radicals.
- **Grapefruit boosts immunity**
  Ingesting grapefruit regularly has been shown to be beneficial for your immune system as it contains high concentrations of vitamin C.
- **You are less likely to get an infection**
  Since vitamin C is an antioxidant, it can boost the protective qualities of the grapefruit and reduce your chances of contracting infections.
- **Grapefruit keeps you hydrated**
  Grapefruit is 90% water and is an ideal food to keep you well hydrated, with hydration being essential for overall body health and cognitive performance.
- **Grapefruit can prevent heart attacks**
  Studies have shown that eating grapefruit daily can help increase the good to bad ratio of cholesterol in your body, helping to reduce the risk for heart attacks and strokes
- **Grapefruit lowers blood pressure**
  It contains high levels of potassium, which is known to neutralise sodium in the body and facilitate a healthy electrolyte balance, lower blood pressure and decrease your risk of hypertension.
- **Grapefruit increases energy**
  The citrus scent of grapefruit is used in aromatherapy to increase your energy, vitality and wake you up.
- **Grapefruit supports cardiac health**
  Several nutrients found in grapefruit, including fibre, lycopene, vitamin C, potassium and choline, are essential for a healthy heart.

Grapes

- **Grapes keep you hydrated**
  Grapes have a high water content that helps to keep your body hydrated and function more effectively.
- **They are good for your kidneys**
  Since grapes have a high water content, it makes it easier for the kidneys to eliminate uric acid.
- **Grapes can boost your immune system**
  Grapes are a great source of vitamins K, A, C and B6, which are all key players in boosting the immune system, decreasing the likelihood of catching colds.
- **Grapes can help prevent cancer**
  Rich in antioxidants, grapes also contain resveratrol, which help reduce damage by free radicals, targeting cancerous and pre-cancerous cells.
- **Grapes can help prevent Alzheimer's**
  They are high in resveratrol, which has been linked to having brain-protecting abilities, such as helping to prevent Alzheimer's disease.
- **They can help with digestion**
  High in fibre, both grapes as raisins can help with digestion and bowel movements, aiding constipation, inflammation and cramps.
- **Grapes can boost your energy levels**
  They are rich in iron, which is a highly important mineral that can treat fatigue and really boost your energy levels.
- **They are good for your heart**
  Grapes contain a healthy dose of potassium, which is believed to drastically reduce your chances, along with a healthy lifestyle, of developing cardiovascular diseases
- **Grapes can help with IBS**
  The anti-inflammatory nature of grapes can help your digestive system quite significantly, having particular benefit to sufferers of IBS and some intolerances.
- **They can help with hayfever**
  Grapes contain quercetin, which is believed to help regulate symptoms of hayfever, relieving sufferers.

Kiwi

- **Kiwis are good for your heart**
  Packed with vitamins, minerals and nutrients, kiwis can contribute greatly towards good cardiovascular health, keeping your heart healthier for longer.
- **They boost your immune system**
  Because of the powerful antioxidants and vitamins found in Kiwis, they effectively boost your immune system, helping you fight illnesses and recover quicker.
- **Kiwis can prevent atherosclerosis**
  It is believed that because of the variety of vitamins and other nutrients found in kiwis, daily consumption can help reduce blood clotting and prevent atherosclerosis.
- **You can sleep better with kiwis**
  Kiwis are a source of serotonin, which promotes less disturbed sleep. Flavanoids present in the fruit modulate sleep-inducing receptors, reducing waking time at night.
- **Kiwis stop you feeling tired**
  The vitamins and phytochemicals found in kiwis help prevent iron deficiencies by increasing iron absorption into the body. This also helps prevent anaemia and fatigue.
- **Kiwis can keep your eyes healthy**
  Kiwis can help protect your eyes from macular degeneration and cataracts, due to their zeaxanthin and lutein content, which are also found in the human eye.
- **They can keep you looking young**
  Kiwi contributes to collagen synthesis with its vitamins. It can be beneficial in wrinkle reduction and the reduction of UV radiation effects.
- **Kiwis help your skin heal quicker**
  Due to the collagen content found in kiwis and their highly nutritional content, they can help abrasions and cuts heal more quickly.
- **They can help reduce the risk of strokes**
  Kiwi seeds are a great source of Omega 3 fatty acids; increasing your intake of Omega 3 can help reduce the risk of stroke
- **Kiwis can help with respiratory difficulties**
  Kiwis have shown protective effects against asthma, greatly decreasing the incidence of wheezing when included in a daily diet.

Lemon

- **Lemons help indigestion**
  Lemon juice can help with indigestion and constipation, as it acts as a blood purifier, easing difficulties with these areas.
- **Lemons can help bad breath**
  A few drops of fresh lemon juice can help to eliminate bad odours in the mouth, helping to reduce bad breath.
- **They can prevent gum bleeding**
  Massaging some fresh lemon juice onto the gums can help prevent bleeding gums and also ease the symptoms of bleeding gums.
- **Lemons soothe toothache**
  As well as helping with bad breath and bleeding gums, it is believed that massaging fresh lemon juice onto the gums of the affected area can also help ease toothache.
- **Lemons are great for sunburn**
  Lemons act as a natural antiseptic and so adding lemon juice to an after sun cream, hydration cream or directly to the skin, can help soothe sunburn and calm the affected area.
- **They can sooth bee stings**
  Because lemon juice is a natural antiseptic, using the juice on infections or inflamed skin can help heal the wound or wounded area; adding lemon juice to a bee sting can help reduce the pain greatly.
- **Lemon juice can clear your skin**
  High in antioxidants and a powerful natural antiseptic, lemon juice can help various skin conditions, including acne and eczema.
- **Lemons can relieve respiratory diseases**
  Lemon juice works to open the air ways and relieve respiratory diseases, including helping to reduce the symptoms of asthma and asthma attacks.
- **Lemons help control heart health**
  Potassium-rich lemons help control blood pressure and nausea, reducing mental stress. Inhaling lemon oil can help increase concentration and alertness.
- **Lemons are good for your cholesterol**
  Pectin found in lemons, along with other nutrients can help lower bad cholesterol in the body.
- **Lemon juice and kidney health**
  Some research suggests lemon juice may support kidney health, potentially protecting against kidney stone development.

Lime

- **Limes can help prevent cancer**
  Limes contain flavonoid and limonoid compounds,which have antioxidant qualities and help destroy free radicals, believed to help target, fight and destroy precancerous and cancerous cells.
- **Limes can prevent cholera**
  Rich in antioxidants, limes have many antibiotic effects and are believed to help protect against cholera.
- **They can help protect against rheumatoid arthritis & osteoarthritis**
  Lies are full of antioxidants and flavanols, which help reduce cell damage. This has the benefit of preventing and easing many diseases and illnesses, including reducing symptoms of rheumatoid arthritis and osteoarthritis.
- **You are less likely to get food poisoning**
  Kaffir limes fight harmful bacteria, such as E. coli, which often causes food poisoning in many foods.
- **Limes can help prevent acne**
  The oil from Kaffir limes can help prevent acne from developing, growing and worsening, as well as helping to heal typical blemishes.
- **Limes help burn fat**
  Citric acid present in limes is great for burning fat, helping you to lose excess weight and manage weight loss in general.
- **They can refresh your palate**
  Limes are believed to cleanse your taste buds and provide a refreshing clean, making them ideal inbetween meals.
- **They can help clean you internally**
  Lime juice is believed to clean and cleanse the excretory system and consequently ease constipation, inflammation and cramps.
- **Limes can help diabetes**
  Limes contain high levels of soluble fibre that help regulate sugar absorption in the body, therefore preventing sugar spikes seen in diabetics.
- **Limes can help prevent heart disease**
  Soluble fibre can also help lower blood pressure and decrease bad cholesterol. This in turn protects the body from heart disease and strokes.
- **They can help treat urinary infections**
  High in potassium, limes are great at removing toxic substances from the body and help to quickly clear up any infections in the urinary system

Mango

- **Mangos can help prevent against cancer**
  High in antioxidants, mangos help the body to fight free radicals which are linked to the development of many cancers.
- **Mango lowers cholesterol**
  Fibre, pectin and vitamin C, all present in mangos, all help lower bad cholesterol in the body, which has many health benefits for the body.
- **Mangos keep the eyes healthy**
  Mango contains vitamin A, crucial in helping our eyesight and preventing dry eye conditions.
- **They can unclog your pores**
  Rich in vitamins and minerals, the combination of these nutrients in mango helps to maintain healthy membranes and skin, and unclog pores that cause spots and acne.
- **Mangos can boost your libido**
  They provide vitamin E that, in balanced amounts, help regulate sex hormones and boost your sex drive.
- **Mangos can help ease for heat stroke**
  Mango juice and water can help to cool down the body following heat stroke, as well as soothing it.
- **They are good for hangovers**
  Mangos help your kidneys excrete toxins and to process quicker, helping the body to recover from alcohol more quickly.
- **Mango is good for memory**
  Due to the glutamine acid, mango is good for concentration and memory. vitamin B6 is vital for good brain function, especially for neurotransmitters, which contribute to sleeping patterns and mood.
- **Mango is good for digestion**
  Mangos can eliminate excess acidity from the digestive system. Esters, terpenes and aldehydes help to enhance appetite and aid indigestion.
- **Mango can be good during pregnancy**
  Full of iron, mangos are a great alternative to iron tablets, which bring along unwanted side effects. This will also help prevent against anaemia and aid fatigue.
- **They boost your immune system**
  Carotenoids found in mangos enhance the immune system, protecting it from bacteria and toxins and helping to fight off the common cold, which strengthens immunity further.

Melon

- **Melons are good for your blood pressure**
  They are rich in potassium, which helps to control blood pressure and heart rate, as well as regulating sodium.
- **They boost the immune system**
  Rich in Vitamin B complex (B1, B3, B5, B6), melons help to protect the immune system and enable it to work as effectively as possible.
- **Melons are good for cholesterol**
  Vitamin B complex, which is great for the immune system, also helps increase good cholesterol and the breakdown of carbohydrates and fats for energy.
- **Melons are good for your eyes**
  As a source of vitamin A, melons help keep your eyes healthy in terms of vision, but are also hydrating, helping to prevent dry eye conditions.
- **Melons make your bones and teeth stronger**
  Due to the high calcium content, melons can help to maintain strong teeth and bones in the body.
- **Melons are great for hydration**
  Melons are 90% water which, along with their potassium content, help to regulate water levels in the body, keeping cells hydrated.
- **They can help reduce the risk and symptoms of diabetes**
  Insulin production has to be regulated in diabetics and melons help with this task; they are low in glucose, further decreasing the risk of diabetes.
- **Melons are good for pregnancy**
  With a weakened immunity, a pregnant body requires additional minerals and nutrients. As well as this, it also provides potassium which helps maintain a healthy heart by lowering blood pressure.
- **They can aid weight loss**
  Due to their high water content, but low calorie content, melon makes a great snack alternative to aid with weight loss and management and suppress cravings.
- **Melons are good for morning sickness**
  Melons contain vitamins A and C, which can help ease nausea and morning sickness, as well as general sickness.

HIDDEN *Healing* POWERS

of

NUTS &
BEANS

Almonds

- **Almonds are good for the heart**
  As a food containing monosaturated fat (good fat!), almonds can help the body maintain and balance its levels of cholesterol, which in turn benefits the heart.
- **They can help your memory**
  Almonds are full of a variety of nutrients that are good for the brain; l-carnitine, which helps to protect our brain, can be found in almonds and it is suggested that it can, in turn, help prevent memory loss.
- **Almonds can help protect against diabetes**
  Almonds help your body to regulate its processing and consequently, absorption of glucose and reduce increases in insulin, benefiting diabetes sufferers, helping to protect against it.
- **Almonds are good for you during pregnancy**
  During pregnancy, women are encouraged to increase their intake of folic acid to help the baby obtain all the right nutrients. Almonds are a good source of folic acid.
  Note: If there is a history of nut allergies in your family, you may be recommended to abstain from consuming nuts during pregnancy; always consult with your doctor first.
- **Almonds can make you feel less hungry.**
  A recent study found that choosing to snack on almonds can reduce cravings and feelings of hunger.
- **Almonds make your skin smoother**
  You can find many alternative skin creams and oils that are made from almonds. This is because they are great for nurturing and hydrating your skin. It is thought that the use of almond oils or creams during pregnancy can reduce a women's chance of stretch marks.
- **They are good for your hair and nails.**
  Almonds, like many other nuts, contain high levels of calcium and phosphorous which helps your hair and nails to grow and remain strong.
- **Almonds boost your immune system**
  Rich in many nutrients, almonds are also considered an alkali food. Since disease struggles to fester in alkaline environments, consuming almonds can help your body fight off illness.
- **Almonds can reduce your risk of heart attacks**
  Vitamin E and magnesium, both found in almonds, have been linked to reducing the risk of a heart attack and heart disease.

Black Beans

- **Black beans keep your sugar levels steady**
  With many foods, as they pass through your body they increase your blood sugar levels. Spikes in sugar levels is not always a good thing and is dangerous for diabetes sufferers. Black beans, however, have a stabilising effect on blood sugar levels.
- **They lower your cholesterol**
  Black beans are rich in nutrients and contain soluble fibre, which is known to bring down your cholesterol
- **They can reduce the risk of cancer of the bowel and colon**
  Black beans contain fatty acids that are good for our intestines when passing through them. These fatty acids are used by cells found in our large intestine to refuel and rejuvenate, which is thought by some to reduce the risk of bowel and colon cancers.
- **They are good for you during pregnancy**
  During pregnancy, women are encouraged to increase their intake of folic acid to help the baby obtain all the right nutrients and aid brain development. Black beans are a rich source of folic acid.
- **Black beans can prevent Parkinson's and Alzheimer's**
  They are rich in folic acid, which helps with brain development. It is believed that low levels of an absence of this nutrient can lead to the onset of Parkinson's and Alzheimer's; and so, increasing your folic acid intake can help prevent these diseases.
- **Black beans boost your health**
  They among only a few foods that naturally contain the mineral molybdenum. Molybdenum essentially works as an activator for enzymes throughout the body, required for our many different health systems.
- **Black beans can help prevent cancer**
  They contain flavonoids in their 'soft shell' or 'outer layer'.
- **They can help your performance in the bedroom**
  Molybdenum, a mineral found in black beans, does not only help activate essential enzymes in your body, but is also believed to increase a man's sex drive and reduce erectile dysfunction.
- **Black beans can prevent osteoporosis**
  Rich in the likes of calcium, magnesium and phosphorous, black beans help to strengthen and maintain the strength of your bones as well as supporting your joints. In turn, this helps to prevent diseases like osteoporosis.

Brazil Nuts

- **Brazil nuts are good for your cholesterol**
  Rich in good fatty acids, brazil nuts contain good cholesterol and can help maintain a balance in your body when consumed in small portions.
- **They are good for bowel movements**
  Since brazil nuts are high in fibre, they can help regulate your bowel movements helping with things like constipation, bloating and cramps.
- **They reduce your risk of a heart attack**
  Brazil nuts help to balance your cholesterol, which is closely associated with a reduced risk of heart attack or stroke.
- **Brazil nuts kick start your metabolism**
  Selenium can be found in brazil nuts and is often known for how it benefits the skin; it also helps our thyroid glands work properly. When our thyroid glands are working properly, our metabolism does too and receives a natural boost.
- **Brazil nuts can stop you ageing**
  Brazil nuts contain selenium, a powerful antioxidant that helps prevent the formation of wrinkles through maintaining the elasticity in your skin
- **You'll heal quicker**
  Brazil nuts help your body to repair and heal itself through cell rejuvenation because of their high protein content. They also provide you with all the essential amino acids, which are crucial for your body to grow and repair.
- **They make your skin glow**
  Brazil nuts are rich in a variety of nutrients that help to keep your skin looking youthful providing you with a healthy glow.
- **Brazil nuts boost your immune system**
  Full of great nutrients, minerals and antioxidants, brazil nuts stimulate the production of white blood cells to boost your immune system and fight off illness.
- **They keep you fuller for longer**
  Brazil nuts, like many other nuts, seeds and lentils, are digested by your body much slower than other foods, which means you are left feeling fuller for longer.

Cashew Nuts

- **Cashew nuts are good for your heart**
  Rich in antioxidants, cashew nuts can help keep your heart healthy.
- **They are good for your nervous system**
  Rich in magnesium, consuming cashew nuts really benefits your nervous system; magnesium works as a barrier for calcium to enter your blood system which can prevent your nervous system from working effectively.
- **They stop you getting gallstones**
  Studies have found that frequently consuming cashew nuts can dramatically reduce your chances of developing gallstones – reports suggest they reduce the risk by as much as 25%.
- **Cashew nuts are good for your bones**
  We commonly associated calcium with bone strength, however magnesium is equally as important. Rich in magnesium, cashew nuts can help strengthen your bones.
- **Cashew nuts help lower blood pressure**
  They contain the important mineral magnesium, which helps lower blood pressure.
- **They are low in fat**
  Unlike many other nuts, cashew nuts have a low fat content, so you can consume a much larger portion to benefit from their goodness without having to worry about high levels of fat or calories.It is commonly known that snacking on nuts can make you feel fuller for longer, reduce cravings and are more likely to stop you from over-eating. Due to their low fat content, cashew nuts can be very effective as a snack replacement in helping you lose weight.
- **They enrich your hair colour**
  Copper, found in cashew nuts, is the important mineral that keeps our hair colour the colour that it is. Consuming foods naturally containing copper, like cashew nuts, can help you develop a richer, stronger hair colour.
- **Cashew Nuts can help prevent cancer**
  Like some other nuts and superfoods, cashews contain something called flavonols. A type of flavonol found in cashew nuts helps the body fight against radicals, such as cancerous cells, potentially reducing and destroying them.

Chia Seeds

- **Chia seeds help your digestion**
  They are rich in fibre, which helps ensure that your digestive system works efficiently and stays healthy.
- **They can help stabilise your blood sugar levels**
  Chia seeds contain a good balance of nutrients, including fibre, fat and protein, these work together to provide a steady release of energy rather than spikes, which helps stabilise your blood sugar levels.
- **Chia seeds can help you heal quicker**
  They are rich in phosporous, important in helping your body repair and renew cells and tissue to keep you healthy and heal quickly.
- **Chia seeds are good for your bones**
  Rich in calcium, chia seeds are good for strengthening your bones and preventing osteoporosis.
- **They keep you fuller for longer**
  Chia seeds, alike many other nuts, seeds and lentils, are full of fibre and are digested much slower than other foods, which means you are left feeling fuller for longer.
- **Chia seeds are great for vegans**
  Chia seeds are full of calcium; they are an excellent source of the mineral and a small portion (25g) actually contains more calcium than a small glass of milk (100ml), making them a great alternative for vegans or intolerance sufferers.
- **Chia seeds are good for diabetes**
  It is thought that by helping with digestion, along with their vast nutrient content, chia seeds can help reduce the blood pressure of diabetes sufferers.
- **They lower your cholesterol**
  Chia seeds are rich in nutrients, protein and fibre and slowly release energy, which is known to bring down your cholesterol.
- **Chia seeds boost your immune system**
  Full of antioxidants, vitamins and minerals, chia seeds stimulate the production of white blood cells to boost your immune system and fight off illness.
- **Chia seeds are great for your skin**
  They are incredibly rich in antioxidants, which help prompt the skin's repair systems and cell rejuvenation, keeping your skin looking fresh and young.

Flax Seeds

- **Flax seeds are good for your heart**
  Rich in good fatty acids, such as Omega 3, which help, along with a balanced diet and exercise, to keep your heart healthy.
- **Flax seeds boost your immune system**
  Full of antioxidants, vitamins and minerals, flax seeds stimulate the production of white blood cells to boost your immune system and fight off illness.
- **Flax seeds can help dry skin**
  Rich in 'good' fats and b-vitamins, flax seeds can help hydrate dry skin or skin conditions such as eczema. The seeds can be consumed or their oil can be used.
- **They can help dry eyes**
  Just as flax seeds can benefit your hair and skin, the 'good' fats and b-vitamins in them can also help maintain healthy eyes and keep them hydrated, particularly beneficial for those who suffer with dry eye.
- **Flax seeds are gluten free**
  Completely free from gluten, flax seeds can be used in cooking to replace other seeds or grains for those with intolerances, whilst still providing a wealth of nutrients.
- **Flax seeds boost your immune system**
  As well as being full of antioxidants, flax seeds contain polyphenols which support the growth of probiotics in the body, helping your body to fight off illnesses quicker and more effectively.
- **Flax seeds can help Crohn's sufferers**
  Flax seds contain ALA and help the digestive system; ALA helps the body to protect the lining of the digestive tract, reducing inflammation of the gut, which can be of great benefit to sufferers of Crohn's.
- **They are good for bowel movements**
  Since flax seeds are high in fibre, they can help regulate your bowel movements helping with things like constipation, bloating and cramps.
- **Flax seeds can help prevent cancer**
  A number of studies link the release of lignans by flax seeds when consumed, which help to balance hormones, to a reduced risk in cancer.

Macademia Nut

- **Macademia nuts are good for your heart**
  Cholesterol-free, macademia nuts contain monosaturated fats, which also reduce cholesterol levels, benefiting your heart.
- **Macademia nuts are good for your brain**
  Copper can be found in macademic nuts which is crucial in maintaining neurotransmissions in the brain, keeping your braining healthy for longer.
- **Macademia nuts make you heal quicker**
  Rich in protein, macademia nuts can help your body maintain health cell growth and repair and protect itself.
- **You may be less likely to break a bone**
  Macademia nuts contain the mineral phosphorous which helps maintain bone health and growth to ensure your bones stay as strong as possible for as long as possible.
- **They are good for bowel movements**
  The high fibre content in macademia nuts can help regulate your bowel movements, helping with things like constipation, bloating and cramps.
- **They can stop you from ageing**
  Macademia nuts are high in palmitoleic fatty acids, the fatty acids that delay the ageing of skin through keeping the skin cells hydrated. This is most effective through applying macademia nut oil.
- **They help you get more from vitamins**
  The fatty acids found in macademia nuts helps your body to efficiently absorb nutrients and vitamins found in foods; you can increase a vitamin intake as much as you like, but if your body it not absorbing them properly, you will not benefit from that vitamin or nutrient.
- **Macademia nuts can help prevent osteoporosis**
  Due to the phosphorous found in macademia nuts, bone and joint health is aided which can help prevent the likes of arthritis and osteoporosis.
- **They boost your immune system**
  Rich in antioxidants, macademia nuts boost your immune system, helping your body to fight off illnesses quicker and more effectively. macademia nuts can prevent Trans Epidermal Water Loss (TEWL). Linoleic acid can be found in Macademia Nuts which prevents TEWL from vulnerable skin tissue.

Mustard Seeds

- **Mustard seeds can help the menopause**
  It is common for women going through menopause to suffer bone loss as a result of the change; mustard seeds are rich in calcium and magnesium that can act as preventatives for this.
- **Mustard seeds clear up a cold**
  They work as effective decongestives, helping to clear up and fight off a common cold.
- **They soothe a sore throat**
  Due to their anti-inflammatory and healing qualities, gargling hot water and mustard seeds is recommended for a cough and sore throat.
- **Mustard seeds can help cure bronchitis**
  In addition to effectively clearing up a sore throat, it is believed that mustard seeds can be used to effectively rid a sufferer of bronchitis.
- **They are great for migraines**
  It is thought that the rich content of Omega 3 in Mustard Seeds can help prevent and ease migraines.
- **Mustard seeds help sinus conditions**
  Through working as a decongestive, and containing high levels of Omega 3 and antioxidants, mustard seeds are believed to greatly ease sinus conditions and sinus-related issues.
- **They can get rid of ringworm**
  Mustard seeds can be made into a paste that can then applied be to the affected area, can help heal ringworm because of the level of antioxidants found in the seeds and their healing and anti-inflammatory qualities.
- **They help ease contact dermatitis**
  Mustard seeds contain antioxidants which help the body to repair and protect itself and is believed to greatly help contact dermatitis sufferers because of its healing abilities
- **Mustard seeds can ease psoriasis**
  Antioxidants and enzyme-activating nutrients found in mustard seeds can reduce inflammation in the body and is believed to aid with psoriasis.
- **Mustard seeds can protect against cancer**
  They are full of flavonoids, which help to identify and destroy free radicals in the body, preventing the development and advancement of cancerous and pre-cancerous cells.

Pumpkin Seeds

- **Pumpkin seeds keep your bones stronger for longer**
  They contain magnesium that helps, along with other minerals, to maintain bone health and growth to ensure your bones stay as strong as possible for longer.
- **Pumpkin seeds are good for your heart**
  Rich in good fatty acids, such as Omega 3, which help, along with a balanced diet and exercise, to keep your heart healthy.
- **They can reduce your cholesterol**
  Pumpkin seeds contain phytosterols, which help to manage and reduce cholesterol levels.
- **Pumpkin seeds are good for diabetes**
  The Omega 3 found in pumpkin seeds can help regulate insulin levels, which can help diabetes sufferers manage their insulin levels and minimise complications, as well as reducing cholesterol.
- **They boost your immune system**
  Rich in antioxidants and zinc, pumpkin seeds provide your immune system with a boost, helping your body to fight off illnesses quicker and more effectively.
- **Pumpkin seeds are good for the prostate**
  The zinc found in pumpkin seeds can help men's health as it is believed that zinc can help treat Benign Prostatic Hyperlasia (BPH) and issues associated with enlarged prostate.
- **They can help your performance in the bedroom**
  Pumpkin seeds contain zinc which is important in men in relation to their sexual functions; an increased intake in zinc can help with any issues including erectile dysfunction.
- **Pumpkin seeds can help Crohn's sufferers**
  Pumpkin seeds contain ALA and help the digestive system; ALA helps the body to protect the lining of the digestive tract, reducing inflammation of the gut, which can be of great benefit to sufferers of Crohn's.
- **Pumpkin seeds can help prevent osteoporosis**
  Because of the phosphorous found in pumpkin seeds, bone and joint health is aided, which can help prevent the likes of arthritis and osteoporosis.
- **Pumpkin seeds can make you sleep better**
  They provide a boost of serotonin and niacin, which both help improve sleep, for a good night's rest.

Sunflower Seeds

- **Sunflower seeds are good for your heart**
  Rich in vitamin E, sunflower seeds help to prevent cardiovascular diseases, manage cholesterol and keep your heart healthy.
- **Sunflower seeds are good for your brain**
  Serotonin can be found in sunflower seeds helping to maintain neurotransmissions in the brain, keeping your braining healthy for longer.
- **They are good for your nervous system**
  Rich in magnesium, sunflower seeds benefit your nervous system; magnesium works as a barrier for calcium entering the blood system, which prevents the nervous system from working effectively.
- **You may be less likely to break a bone**
  Sunflower seeds contain high levels of magnesium which, along with calcium, help maintain bone health and growth to ensure your bones stay as strong as possible for as long as possible.
- **Sunflower seeds protect your skin**
  Vitamin E found in sunflower seeds is known to help protect skin against the sun and its UV rays.
- **They can help ease asthma**
  Working as a powerful anti-inflammatory, sunflower seeds can help relieve the symptoms of asthma.
- **They can help relieve osteoarthitis and rheumatoid arthritis**
  Just how pumpkin seeds can help relieve the symptoms of asthma, its anti-inflammatory qualities also help ease the sufferings of osteoarthritis and rheumatoid arthritis.
- **Pumpkin seeds can help prevent osteoporosis**
  Because of the magnesium found in pumpkin seeds, bone and joint health is aided which can help prevent the likes of arthritis and osteoporosis.
- **Sunflower seeds can keep your joints well-oiled**
  In addition to magnesium, which improves durability of bones and joints, copper found in sunflower seeds helps provide and maintain strength and flexibility in joints.
- **Sunflower seeds can help prevent cancer**
  They are full of selenium, which is believed to help prevent the development of cancerous and pre-cancerous cells, as well as identifying and destroying free radicals in the body.

Walnuts

- **Walnuts are good for the heart**
  Walnuts contain ALA, linked to a reduced risk of heart disease.
- **They can reduce your blood pressure**
  Rich in Omega 3, walnuts have been found to increase 'good' cholesterol, whilst reducing 'bad' cholesterol, helping to lower blood pressure.
- **Walnuts are good for your brain**
  They are rich in nutrients, such as vitamin E, Omega 3 and powerful antioxidants, which help general brain health and transmissions, keeping your braining healthy for longer.
- **They boost your immune system**
  Rich in antioxidants, walnuts can help your immune system to operate efficiently, giving it a boost from the enhancing nutrients.
- **They can help ease asthma**
  Working as a powerful anti-inflammatory and high in fatty acids, walnuts can help relieve the symptoms of asthma.
- **They can help relieve eczema**
  In very much the same way that walnuts ease asthma, their anti-inflammatory quality and high fatty acid content helps to calm and reduce eczema and relieve sufferers of the symptoms.
- **Walnuts help your sperm**
  Studies have found that consuming walnuts can positively impact a man's fertility, improving the quality of his sperm if eaten on a daily basis.
- **Walnuts are good for you during pregnancy**
  During pregnancy, women are encouraged to increase their intake of folic acid to help the baby obtain all the right nutrients. Walnuts are a good source of folic acid.
  Note: If there is a history or nut allergy within your family, you may be recommended to abstain from consuming nuts during pregnancy; always consult with your doctor first.
- **Walnuts can help you sleep better**
  Melatonin, found in walnuts, is understood to benefit your sleep and sleeping patterns.
- **Walnuts can help prevent cancer**
  Studies on the consumption of walnuts have suggested that they can reduce the growth of tumours and cancerous growths.

HIDDEN *Healing* POWERS

of

HERBS

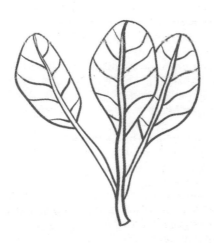

Basil

- **Basil reduces stress**
  Basil is a natural adaptogen, a compound that helps the body rebalance the harmful effects of stress.
- **Basil can regulate our systems**
  The compound adaptogen, found in basil, helps the body to restore the healthy function of numerous body systems, including both the cardiovascular and respiratory systems.
- **Basil helps fight disease**
  Basil contains two powerful antioxidants, viceninare and orientin, which fight damage caused by free radicals and also protect white blood cells involved in the immune response.
- **Basil can help the body self-heal**
  The antibacterial qualities of basil can help the body to heal cuts, wounds, sores and ulcers much more efficiently.
- **Basil may protect against cancer**
  Evidence suggested that the phytochemicals found in basil have cancer preventative properties as they can cause cancer cell death and prevent tumour cells from spreading.
- **Basil can aid IBS**
  Several essential oils found in basil, such as citronellol, eugenol and linalool, reduce inflammation and may lower the risk of inflammatory diseases, including arthritis and IBS.
- **Basil is good for your heart**
  Rich in Vitamin A, basil is believed to protect cells found in blood vessels, helping the flow and transportation of blood around the body. This helps to prevent the build-up of cholesterol and lower the risk of cardiac diseases and stroke.
- **Basil is an anti-diabetic**
  Extracts of basil are low on the glycemic Index and have been shown to reduce sugar levels in the blood and aid the maintenance of healthy blood sugar levels, suggesting a potential treatment for diabetes.
- **Basil helps relieve respiratory diseases**
  Studies have shown that the fresh flowers of basil are effective in treating respiratory conditions, including bronchitis, due to their antioxidant and antimicrobial properties.

Cinnamon

- **Cinnamon is an anti-diabetic**
  Cinnamon has anti-diabetic effects, which can be of great relief to sufferers as it reduces sugar levels in the blood and can promote insulin sensitivity.

- **Cinnamon can prevent tooth decay**
  In addition to preventing bad breath, nutrients in cinnamon are believed to fight off the bacteria found in our mouths to protect against the formation and development of cavities, infections and tooth decay.

- **Cinnamon boosts cognitive function**
  The presence of numerous antioxidants in cinnamon means that is has neuroprotective properties, and through activating proteins helps protects cells from mutation, damage and inflammation, thus lowering the risk of neurodegeneration.

- **Cinnamon may treat candida**
  Cinnamon has powerful anti-fungal properties that have been shown to be effective at preventing candida from overgrowth in the gut, which reduces the risk of the associated autoimmune and digestive symptoms.

- **Cinnamon helps lower cholesterol**
  Evidence suggests that ingesting cinnamon regularly can reduce the levels of bad cholesterol in your blood and reduce your risk of type II diabetes and cardiovascular diseases.

- **Cinnamon may prevent cancer**
  It has been shown that cinnamon extracts can cause cancer cell death and slow the growth of cancerous cells, which may potentially aid in treating some types of cancer.

- **Cinnamon boosts the immune system**
  Cinnamon naturally contains many antibiotic, antifungal and antimicrobial agents, all of which can boost your immune system and help the body fight against toxins and pathogens, reducing your risk of infection.

- **Cinnamon can relieve allergies**
  As an anti-inflammatory, cinnamon has the ability to reduce inflammation and counteract histamine reactions, caused by a variety of allergies. It is therefore considered a natural anti-allergenic, which could reduce the symptoms for allergies and asthma attacks.

Coriander

- **Coriander is good for food poisoning**
  Coriander naturally has antibacterial properties as it contains dodecanal, and evidence shows that it may help the body in fighting off salmonella, the bacteria that causes the symptoms associated with food poisoning.
- **Coriander helps reduce your blood sugar levels**
  Both the essential oil and seeds of coriander have been shown to lower blood sugar levels and increase insulin sensitivity, so may naturally be a treatment for diabetes.
- **Coriander is good for the brain**
  Research has shown that foods high in antioxidants, such as coriander, fight the chronic neuro-inflammation that is associated with age-related cognitive decline and neurological diseases.
- **Coriander is great for your memory**
  High in antioxidants, amongst other nutrients, coriander is believed to help improve the memory and concentration function of the brain.
- **Coriander is good for the menstrual cycle**
  Studies suggest that coriander helps support the endocrine system and maintain normal levels of menstrual hormones, in addition to reducing the negative symptoms such as cramps and bloating.
- **Coriander can relieve pain**
  Extract from coriander seeds has been shown to significantly reduce the feeling of pain in rodents, as it has both analgesic and anti-inflammatory properties; it is thought the same effects can apply to humans.
- **Coriander is great for detoxification**
  Coriander contains antioxidants and studies suggest that coriander extract can prevent lead accumulation due to its antimicrobial and heavy metal chelation properties.
- **Coriander improves your skin**
  Coriander has detoxifying, antiseptic and antioxidant properties, all of which make it the ideal food to hydrate the skin and clear up infections or irritation.
- **Coriander helps lower cholesterol**
  Coriander contains several acidic compounds, including oleic acid, ascorbic acid, and palmitic acid, which have all been shown to lower the levels of bad cholesterol in the blood.

Cumin

- **Cumin can relieve asthma**
  Thymoquione is a compound found in cumin seeds, which has been shown to reduce inflammation of the respiratory tract and effectively ease the symptoms of asthma.
- **Cumin can relieve eczema**
  Rich in vitamin E, cumin has many benefits for our skin and direct application of it onto affected skin areas can help heal skin irritation and eczema.
- **Cumin can help weight loss**
  Studies have shown that an adequate intake of cumin can increase weight loss in individuals and also decrease levels of body fat.
- **Cumin can prevent boils**
  Cumin is great at detoxifying the body because of the cuminaldehyde and thymol compounds found in them, along with phosphorous. Regularly adding cumin to your foods can help prevent the development and growth of boils and spots.
- **Cumin aids digestion**
  It has been shown to increase enzyme activity in the gut and stimulate the release of bile from the liver, both of which are crucial in the digestive process.
- **Cumin can combat anaemia**
  Ingesting foods high in iron, such as cumin, are essential in boosting blood iron levels and increasing red blood cell production, which combat the negative symptoms of anaemia.
- **Cumin can help addiction**
  Several studies in mice have shown that compounds found in cumin can reduce both addictive behaviours and withdrawal symptoms, however the exact compound is not yet known.
- **Cumin can keep your skin clear**
  Cuminaldehyde, found in cumin, is known to help keep your skin clear through its detoxifying and anti-inflammatory properties.
- **Cumin prevents hair loss**
  Black cumin has been shown to fight the thinning of hair, hair falling out, and baldness due to its antioxidant and stimulatory properties.
- **Cumin is anti-ageing**
  Rich in vitamin E, cumin can prolong the effects of ageing on our skin, keeping a healthy, glowing appearance and preventing early formation of wrinkles and sagging skin.

Dill

- **Dill aids digestion**
  Compounds found in dill, along with its fibre content, can help to improve digestion, easing stomach cramps and aches and regulate bowel movements.
- **Dill can prevent bad breath**
  The compounds found in dill can help control oral odours, helping reduce bad breath and keep you fresh.
- **Dill can prevent acid reflux**
  Because dill helps the digestive system and to regulate systems, its nutrients also help to minimise and ease acid reflux.
- **Dill can improve sleeping**
  Dill may be useful in fighting insomnia. Flavanoids and vitamin B complex activate enzymes, which help you have a good night's sleep, provide a calming effect.
- **Dill can reduce bloating**
  Dill is a carminative and can help eliminate excessive gas. It helps gases travel through the digestive tract, leaving the body safely.
- **Dill boosts your immune system**
  Dill has shown anti-microbial properties, able to prevent infections throughout the body.
- **Dill can help your body heal**
  Because of its anti-microbial properties, dill can help the body heal small wounds, cuts and grazes more effectively, enabling the skin to repair and renew quicker.
- **Dill can prevent bad breath**
  Dill seeds and leaves can help refresh your breath. The essential oils also work as disinfectants and antioxidants, minimising gum and tooth damage and disease.
- **Dill can prevent cancer**
  Dill compounds are good at neutralising carcinogens and free radicals. Monoterpenes in dill activate enzymes which help to protect the developments of cancerous and pre-cancerous cells.
- **Dill is good for your bones**
  Rich in calcium; dill is a great source for building and maintaining bone strength to support the body better. An increased intake if calcium can help prevent the likes of osteoporosis.

Fennel

- **Fennel protects against ageing**
  Fennel is rich in vitamins, including B and C, which promote collagen synthesis, helping to maintain healthy skin and prolong the effects of ageing.
- **Fennel can treat colic in babies**
  Fennel is good for treating baby colic. If breastfeeding, mothers can drink fennel tea, which will help to calm the digestive tract and relieve symptoms of colic. It helps prevent the formation of gas.
- **Fennel can reduce menstrual cramps**
  It helps to relax muscles and provides the body with antioxidants, as well having as anti inflammatory and antispasmodic benefits.
  NOTE: Whilst muscles relaxing can ease pain and cramping, as muscles do relax, bleeding can be increased.
- **Fennel can help prevent osteoporosis**
  Fennel bulbs are filled with zinc, iron, phosphorous, calcium, magnesium, manganese and vitamin K. All of these contribute to good bone strength and health. It works by reducing osteoclasts, in turn decreasing weakness in bones.
- **Fennel can help prevent cancer**
  Fennel extracts can inhibit the growth of tumours thanks to flavonoids, alkaloids and phenols.
- **Fennel can help with radiation**
  The flavonoids, alkaloids and phenols found in fennel that help prevent cancer, can also help reduce some if the side effects of radiation during treatment.
- **Fennel is good for the heart**
  Fibre in fennel helps to lower cholesterol in the blood, which helps to decrease the risk of heart disease. Potassium, folate and various vitamins also support the heart. Vitamin B6 and folate help prevent blood vessel damage.
- **Fennel relieves water retention**
  Fennel tea works as a diuretic and helps flush out excess fluids, also helping prevent urinary tract problems.
- **Fennel can reduce puffiness**
  Rich in antioxidants, fennel is an anti-inflammatory; applying fennel tea bags to eyes or swollen areas of the face can reduce puffiness.

Garlic

- **Garlic helps combat sickness**
  Garlic contains allicin, which is a sulphur-containing compound. It has anti-bacterial and anti-fungal properties and helps to flush out toxins. It can also help cure toothache if applied over time.
- **Garlic boosts your immune system**
  Garlic contains vitamins B1, B2, B3, B6, C, calcium, iron, magnesium, manganese, phosphorous, potassium, sodium and zinc. These help to boost the immune system and prevent colds.
- **Garlic can help reduce the risk of heart disease**
  Garlic helps to lower cholesterol levels due to allicin. It also helps to regulate blood sugar levels and blood pressure. It is important to consume garlic raw or semi-cooked for most benefits.
- **Garlic can help prevent cancer**
  Research has shown that garlic boosts the production of hydrogen sulphide, which is believed to help prevent a variety of cancers (prostate, breast, colon).
- **Garlic can help earache**
  It is suggested that adding garlic to a drink can help relieve the symptoms of earache.
- **Garlic can clear the nose**
  It works as a decongestive and either inhaling the steam of garlic in boiling water, or adding garlic to a drink, can help nasal congestion and the common cold.
- **Garlic can get rid of warts**
  Rubbing raw garlic onto the affects area or specific wart, can help reduce the wart and the skin begin to repair and rejuvenate.
- **Antioxidants for dementia**
  Garlic contains antioxidants, which help to clear free radicals in the body, protecting the bod from oxidative damage. Garlic can help increase enzyme activity in the body, and all combined could help prevent common brain diseases, such as dementia.
- **Bones**
  Rodent studies have shown that garlic can increase oestrogen in females and minimise bone loss. This suggests garlic may have positive effects on bone health and osteoarthritis in women.
- **Diabetes**
  Garlic could help diabetics, as it regulates blood sugar levels through enhancement of insulin levels in the blood.

Ginger

- **Ginger can help motion sickness**
  Ginger seems to show positive effects on motion sickness. In one study of naval cadets, those that consumed ginger powder showed less serious symptoms.
- **Ginger can help morning sickness**
  Just as ginger can aid sufferers of motion sickness, it can also help ease the symptoms of morning sickness. Ginger drinks or ginger biscuits are a common 'turn to'.
- **Ginger helps your circulation**
  Chromium, magnesium and zinc help to improve the blood flow, helping to prevent the likes of chilblains often caused by poor circulation.
- **Ginger can reduce sweating**
  By regulating the blood flow around your body, consuming ginger can in turn help regulate chills, fever or sweating, especially if excessive.
- **Ginger can help clear a cold**
  Ginger has been used as a natural treatment for thousands of years for the common cold or flu. It is commonly used within a tea.
- **Ginger can reduce stomach ache**
  Ginger aids digestion and improves food absorption. It also helps to reduce inflammation, slightly like aspirin or ibuprofen. It also helps combat morning sickness, showing a 75% success rate.
- **Ginger helps you digest and absorb**
  Ginger helps to aid digestion and improve nutrient absorption, by regulating metabolism.
- **Ginger can help prevent cancer**
  Results from mice studies show potential for ginger in delaying the growth of colorectal and ovarian cancer cells.
- **Ginger can kill off fungus**
  Garlic extract is the most effective at killing fungus; out of 29 plan species evaluated. Shagelol and gingerol are the most active compounds for this condition.
- **Ginger can remedy headaches**
  By rubbing Ginger into the affected area, such as your temples if suffering with a headache, it is commonly reported that ginger dramatically eases the symptoms of headaches, even for regular sufferers.

Lemon Balm & Mint

- **Lemon balm & mint help you heal**
  Caffeic acid and rosmarinic acid help to neutralise free radicals. They have antibacterial and antiviral properties and help to protect cells.
- **They can aid relaxation**
  Lemon balm oil is very expensive and is actively used in aromatherapy; the oil has an uplifting and calming effect on our senses.
- **Lemon balm can relive stress**
  Lemon balm can help increase the body's resistance to stress, building resilience and having a more calming effect.
- **Lemon balm & mint can heal cold sores**
  The soothing and antioxidant qualities can help treat the likes of cold sores and ulcers when applied directly to the affected area.
- **They can help restful sleep**
  The calming effect of lemon balm & mint can help you fall asleep more easily, as well as sleep better to ensure that you are much more rested.
- **They can improve memory**
  Lemon balm can help improve problem solving and memory for both young and old. A phytochemical in the balm suppresses the breakdown of memory relevant neurotransmitter.
- **They are good for your liver**
  Antioxidants glutathione and superoxide dismutase are very important for good liver health. Lemon balm supports the production of these compounds.
- **They are good for your digestion**
  Lemon balm & mint stimulate the digestive system, helping deal with cramps, nausea, diarrhoea and constipation.
- **Mint can help colic in babies**
  It is believed that mint can help calm babies suffering with colic; either through the use of oils, or the mother, if breastfeeding, through drinking mint or peppermint tea.
- **They aid respiration**
  Lemon balm and mint contain very powerful compounds, which can help alleviate symptoms of many common health issues. The aromas can help clear up congestion, beneficial for asthma sufferers.

Mustard Seeds

- **Mustard seeds can help fight cancer**
  Rich in phytonutrients, mustard seeds show the potential to stimulate tumour cell death. Similar studies have also shown inhibition of bladder cancer cell growth.
- **Mustard seeds can aid thyroid regulation**
  Selenium is a mineral which helps clear free radicals and is responsible for the transformation of T4 hormone into T3, a more active form. This helps to maintain thyroid function.
- **They can aid IBS**
  Mustard seeds are an anti-inflammatory, packed with nutrients which help reduce inflammation in the body and relieve IBS symptoms as well as other digestive issues.
- **Mustard seeds can relieve symptoms of rheumatoid arthritis**
  curcuminoids, which actually give mustard its yellow colour, has healing and soothing properties and can be used to ease pain from conditions like rheumatoid arthritis.
- **Mustard seeds are good for digestion**
  Antiseptic and antifungal properties of mustard seeds help to clean and cleanse the digestive system, relieving the symptoms of constipation, diarrhoea, cramps and inflammation.
- **They are good for your immune system**
  Filled with antioxidants and antiseptic properties, mustard seeds are great for giving your immune system a well needed boost.
- **Mustard seeds help respiration**
  Mustard seeds are very good at helping with pneumonia and bronchitis. Direct application to the chest and throat can help decrease symptoms of respiration related diseases.
- **Mustard seeds can combat anaemia**
  Mustard seeds are rich in copper, iron, magnesium and selenium, which can naturally boost the body's iron and energy levels to help fight against anaemia.
- **Mustard seeds boost the immune system**
  As a source of dietary fibre, the seeds improve digestion and metabolism in the body. It is effective as it is soluble and can be used by the body easily.
- **They are good for your skin**
  Mustard seeds help to hydrate and detoxify your skin.

Oregano

- **Oregano boosts your immune system**
  Oregano contains many nutrients such as potassium, zinc, iron and calcium, as well as fibre and magnesium, which all contribute to boosting your immune system.
- **Oregano is good for your gums**
  Oregano helps protect cell deterioration, helps form collagen and holds cells together, maintaining your teeth and keeping your gums healthy.
- **Oregano can prevent infections**
  Full of minerals, oregano has been shown to help prevent and fight against many fungal and bacterial infections in the body and on the skin.
- **Oregano can help your gut**
  High in fibre; oregano can help maintain a healthy digestive system, helping move food through the digestive tract. It also helps improve nutrient absorption and a healthy gut
- **Oregano is good for your bones**
  Calcium, iron and manganese, amongst other minerals found in oregano, can help maintain your bone and joint strength, helping to protect against the like of osteoporosis.
- **Oregano can make you look more youthful**
  Oregano can have anti-ageing qualities, which help protect cell deterioration and aid the formation of collagen, helping to keep a youthful look about your skin.
- **Oregano aids circulation**
  Oregano is rich in B vitamins, which help to rejuvenate the body through increased circulation. Iron and increased haemoglobin deliver more oxygen to the cells in the body, increasing energy.
- **Oregano boosts your energy levels**
  The variety of nutrients and minerals found in oregano do not only boost your immune system, but also naturally increase your energy levels.
- **Oregano is good for your heart**
  Oregano contains Omega-3 fatty acids, which help rebalance cholesterol levels and prevent atherosclerosis, heart attacks and strokes.

Parsley

- **Parsley boosts your immune system**
  Rich in Vitamin K and C, parsley gives your immune system a natural boost to help fight off common illnesses and diseases.
- **Parsley is good for your bones**
  Packed with vitamin C, parsley helps with maintaining bone health and strength, as well as that of your joints.
- **Parsley keeps you healthy**
  Rich in antioxidants, parsley is one of the most anti-oxidising plants known to man, and helps to fight free radicals, keeping you, along with a healthy lifestyle, healthier for longer.
- **It can relieve joint pain**
  Due to the anti-inflammatory properties of parsley; daily use of the herb can help relieve joint pain.
- **Parsley helps fatigue**
  High in iron, parsley can help treat anaemia. Healthy levels of iron help to increase oxygen in the blood, also increasing energy levels.
- **Parsley can help diabetes**
  Parsley can help prevent and treat diabetes through the nutrient myricetin. Another compound found in parsley called flavonol also helps to reduce incidence of diabetes.
- **Parsley can help prevent cancer**
  Flavonoids help to clear the body of disease-causing agents. Flavanoids in parsley can help to prevent skin cancer and block cancer-causing effects of amines. Apigenin, also found in parsley, has been shown to decrease tumour size in breast cancer.
- **Parsley is good for your gums**
  Eugenol can be found in parsley which is frequently used as an antiseptic to help treat gum diseases and mouth ulcers.
  NOTES: Be aware that the use of Eugenol can reduce blood sugar levels.
- **Parsley can aid indigestion**
  The anti-inflammatory, healing and anti-oxidising properties of parsley can help relieve the symptoms of indigestion.
- **Parsley is good during pregnancy**
  Parsley is a great source of calcium and folic acid, vital during pregnancy for the development of the foetus.

Rosemary

- **Rosemary can fight infections**
  The herb contains rosmarinic acid and essential oils, which have anti-inflammatory, antiseptic and anti-fungal properties, helping the body to fight off infections.

- **Rosemary can help prevent cancer**
  Manganese and other minerals support the body in fighting free radicals. This helps to lower the risk of cancer and studies have shown the power of these compounds in helping breast cancer patients.

- **Rosemary can boost energy levels**
  Rich in iron, rosemary can provide a natural increase in energy levels, helping combat tiredness and fatigue.

- **Rosemary can help manage blood pressure**
  Iron and potassium can both be found in rosemary and are both involved in the regulation of blood pressure, heart rate and blood oxygen.

- **Rosemary can help you concentrate**
  Improved concentration has been noted through the consumption of rosemary, due to increased blood flow to the heart and brain.

- **Rosemary can help depression**
  Since rosemary increases the blood flow around the body, heart and brain, it can be a useful treatment for depression or mental fatigue, as well as help alleviate some symptoms of neurodegenerative disorders.

- **Rosemary can aid respiration**
  Rosemary oil is effective in the relief of congestion and minor respiratory struggles, such as common cough and colds.

- **Rosemary can help allergies**
  Rosemary oil can also offer relief for allergy sufferers, in particular hayfever, through acting as a decongestive and working as an antiseptic with anti-inflammatory properties.

- **Rosemary is good for indigestion**
  Rosemary can also help eliminate stomach cramps and gas. It stimulates bile production by the gall bladder, aiding in digestion, especially of meats.

- **Rosemary can help bad breath**
  Rosemary can simply be used to eliminate mouth odours, by helping to clear oral bacteria as well as preventing cavities or plaque.

Sage

- **Sage can help oily skin**
  Sage helps regulates the production of sebum, a fatty secretion from glands, which aids the production of oils in our skin; an increase of sage can help manage these levels.
- **Sage can make your hair grow**
  Rich in nutrients and hydrating qualities, sage can help to stimulate hair growth and prevent hair loss, especially if applied directly to the scalp.
- **Sage can reduce sweating**
  Sage extract or an infusion of the herb can reduce sweating by up to 50%, eliminate associated odours and dry perspiration.
- **Sage is good for indigestion**
  It can help to treat weaknesses in the digestive system. Teas or infusions can help remove symptoms of indigestion, as well as improve bile flow and intestinal mobility and function.
- **Sage can help heal a sore throat**
  Sage is good for the treatment of throat infections and ulcers because of its anti-inflammatory and healing qualities; it is most effective when gargled as a solution.
- **Sage is good for the brain**
  Sage essential oil affects the levels of acetylcholinesterase, which is an enzyme crucial in production of neurotransmitters, keeping your brain sharper for longer.
- **Sage is good for your memory**
  It contains the neurotransmitter acetylcholine, which is important for maintaining memory capacity, improving memory and improving concentration levels.
- **Sage can prevent cardiovascular diseases**
  The flavone salvigenin found in sage can help protect against cardiovascular disease as it the compound can act as a vascular relaxant.
- **Sage can help depression**
  Thujone is a compound found in sage, which is known to block GABA and serotonin receptors, in turn alleviating symptoms of depression, improving concentration and attention span.

Thyme

- **Thyme can help lower blood pressure**
  Thyme has the ability to reduce high blood pressure and lower cholesterol.
- **Thyme can cure the common cold**
  Oil obtained from leaves of thyme can be used to help your body to fight off the common cough and cold.
- **Thyme is good for respiration**
  Due to its healing qualities and decongestive properties, thyme can help respiratory conditions, such as acute bronchitis.
- **Thyme can make you feel happy**
  Carvacrol is an active substance found in thyme that affects our neuron activities. It improves the feeling of wellbeing and is often used for therapeutic purposes.
- **Thyme can help fight infection**
  Rich in antioxidants, thyme can help to protect the body from free radicals, by identifying them and stimulating the destruction of these cells and changes in them.
- **Thyme can prevent ageing**
  The high levels of antioxidants in thyme can help prolong the effects of ageing on the skin, such as wrinkle formation.
- **Thyme can help the reproductive system**
  As well as helping to fight infections in our digestive and respiratory systems, the antioxidants in thyme can also help to fight some infections of the reproductive system.
- **Thyme is good for indigestion**
  Tea made from fresh thyme leaves can help provide relief from gas and bloating. Oils found in thyme can also help cure intestinal cramping.
- **Thyme can combat anaemia**
  As a source of iron, thyme can help stimulate red blood cells and improve energy production. This will also help prevent fatigue and boost the immune system.
- **Thyme is a sleep remedy**
  Thyme tea with honey can help induce sound sleep and keep nightmares away. It also shows calming effects, at the same time reducing tiredness.

Turmeric

- **Turmeric is good for the brain**
  Research has shown turmeric can induce cell death in brain tumours.
  It could also have effects against cancers which are resistant to other
  forms of treatment.
- **Turmeric can help prevent cancer**
  Curcumin, the yellow compound found in turmeric, has positive effects
  on melanoma cells, which can help prevent the development of
  cancerous and pre-cancerous cells.
- **Turmeric can help chemotherapy**
  Curcumin also helps enhance a chemotherapy treatment using
  cisplatin. Together they are better at suppressing tumours.
- **Turmeric can help side effects of chemotherapy**
  Not only does turmeric help the efficiency of chemotherapy, but the
  compound found in turmeric, curcumin, also helps to protect healthy
  cells from the toxic effects.
- **Turmeric keeps your eyes healthy**
  Curcumin may be effective in treating some types of degenerative
  eye diseases. This can help to prevent blindness and also help treat
  macular degeneration.
- **Turmeric can aid weight loss**
  Curcumin in turmeric reduces leptin resistance and activates the fat
  burning processes, helping you to lose excess weight and manage
  weight.
- **Turmeric can reduce blood sugar levels**
  Curcumin is an incredibly useful compound in turmeric; it also lowers
  the body's insulin resistance and can help to reverse hyperglycaemia.
- **Turmeric is good for the liver**
  Tumeric helps to detoxify the liver and protect it from liver damage,
  for example, damage caused by the consumption of excessive alcohol
  or a high fat diet.
- **Turmeric may help prevent MS**
  Multiple sclerosis incidence is much lower in India and China, where
  turmeric is consumed on a daily basis. Curcumin is believed to slow the
  progression of the disease.
- **Turmeric can help depression**
  Curcumin may help prevent and relieve major depression; a study
  showed participants that took Prozac along with curcumin showed
  better results than each by itself.

Food Diary

Many of us suffer from food intolerances, indeed, the number of people who believe they suffer from these has dramatically risen in recent years, according the NHS.

A food intolerance is when the body has difficulty digesting certain foods and has a disagreeable reaction to that particular food. For example, bloating, stomach pain and diarrhoea are symptoms, as well as skin reactions. A food allergy is different, as it involves your immune system reacting to certain foods and triggering symptoms, such as rash or wheezing and can be serious.

If you suffer from symptoms that may suggest you have an intolerance (such as lactose, wheat or gluten) the only real way to get to the root cause is to keep an accurate and regular record of what you eat. Symptoms of intolerances normally would appear a few hours after eating (allergic reactions are much quicker), so keeping a diary of your food intake can help you discover what may be causing the problem. Bear in mind the problem could also be in caffeine, alcohol or artificial preservatives, to name just a few.

On the following pages is a simple 4 week food diary for you to keep. Every day note which foods you eat, how much, the time of day and when symptoms appear. Try to include as much detail as you can including any sauces or condiments that you may have used when making your meal. Also include all drinks and snacks.

Over a period of least 4 weeks you should be able to start pinpointing some possible culprits. Moving forward, try eliminating these foods from your diet one by one and noting if this has any positive effect on your symptoms. Ideally you should keep them eliminated for at least 2-3 weeks. If you do find an improvement after removing a food, try reintroducing what you believe to be the offending ingredient to confirm it is indeed the cause. It may be necessary to keep a food diary for a number of months before identifying what may be causing your symptoms.

Food diaries are a great way of examining your diet. Even if you do not suffer from any intolerances or allergies it can be a helpful way to analyse your nutrition and look for ways to introduce healthier fruit, veg, nuts, beans and herbs and all their potential benefits listed in this book.

If you have severe symptoms or are in any way concerned we recommend you seek advice from your GP or a dietician.

Food & Liquid	Amount of Food or Liquid	Time Food or Liquid Eaten	Time Symptoms Begin	Symptom Description	Remarks
MON e.g. brown toast & butter. cup of tea with whole milk & 1 sweetener	1 slice 1 cup	8.15am	9.30am	dull tummy ache	
TUE					
WED					

THUR | FRI | SAT | SUN

Food & Liquid	Amount of Food or Liquid	Time Food or Liquid Eaten	Time Symptoms Begin	Symptom Description	Remarks
MON					
TUE					
WED					

SUN	SAT	FRI	THUR

Food & Liquid	Amount of Food or Liquid	Time Food or Liquid Eaten	Time Symptoms Begin	Symptom Description	Remarks
MON					
TUE					
WED					

| THUR | FRI | SAT | SUN |

Food & Liquid	Amount of Food or Liquid	Time Food or Liquid Eaten	Time Symptoms Begin	Symptom Description	Remarks
MON					
TUE					
WED					

THUR	FRI	SAT	SUN

If you enjoyed

— HIDDEN *Healing* POWERS —

of

SUPER & WHOLE

FOODS

you may also enjoy other books from CookNation including:

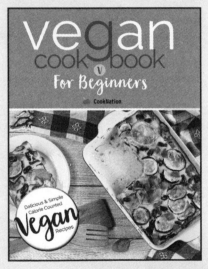

To browse the full catalogue visit
www.bellmackenzie.com

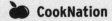